# Snake Venom and Ecology

*Edited by Mohammad Manjur Shah,
Umar Sharif, Tijjani Rufai Buhari
and Tijjani Sabiu Imam*

Published in London, United Kingdom

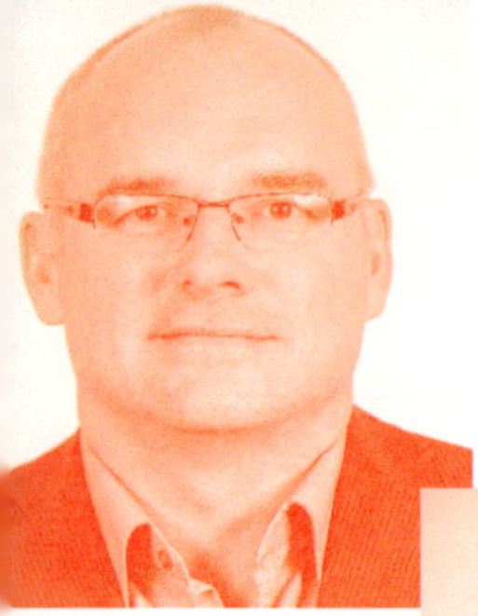
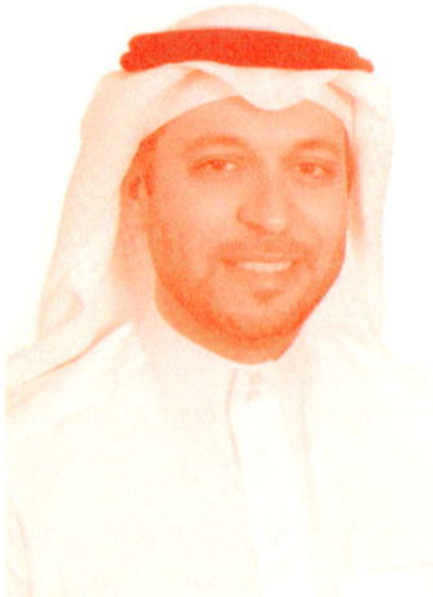
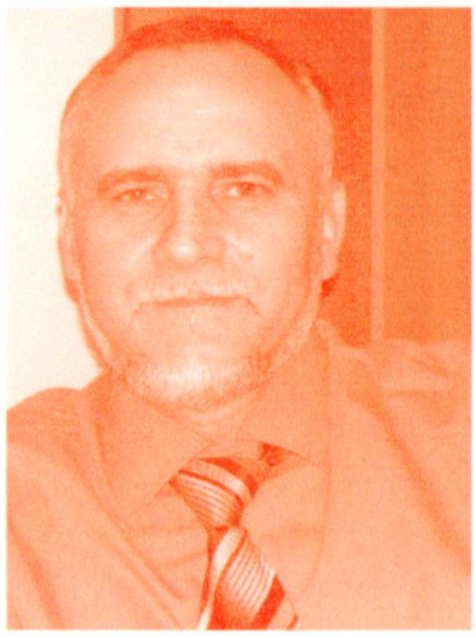
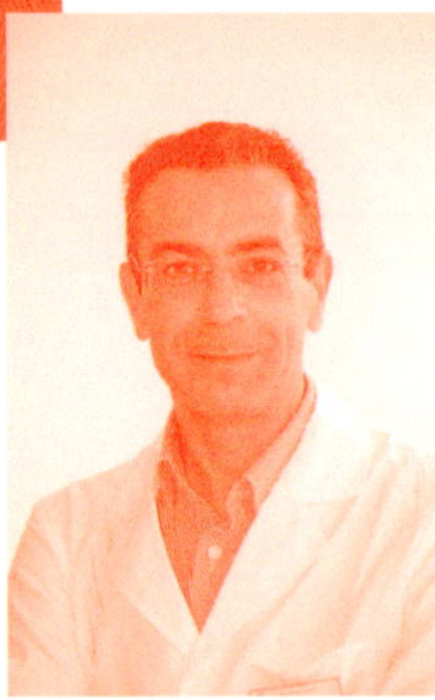
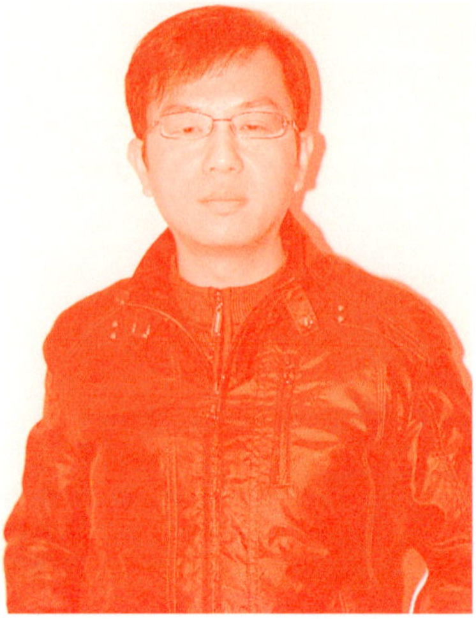
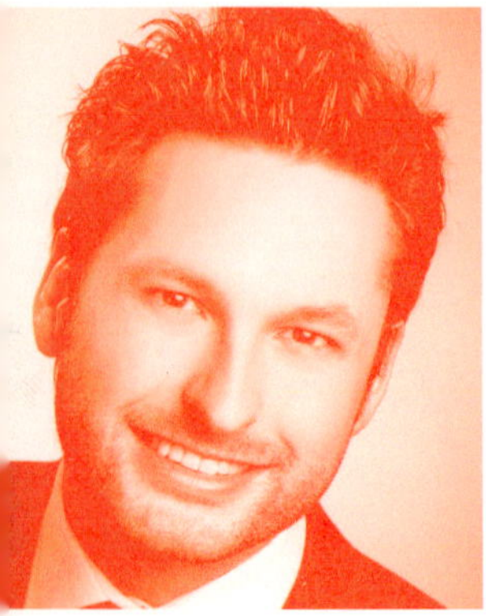
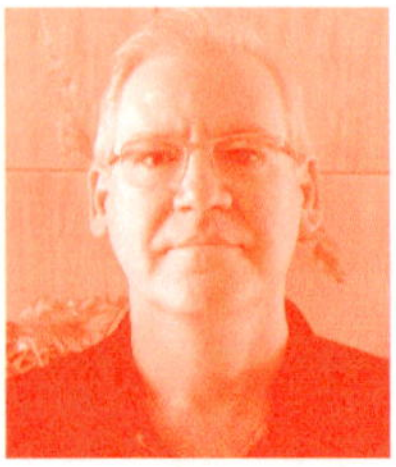

IntechOpen

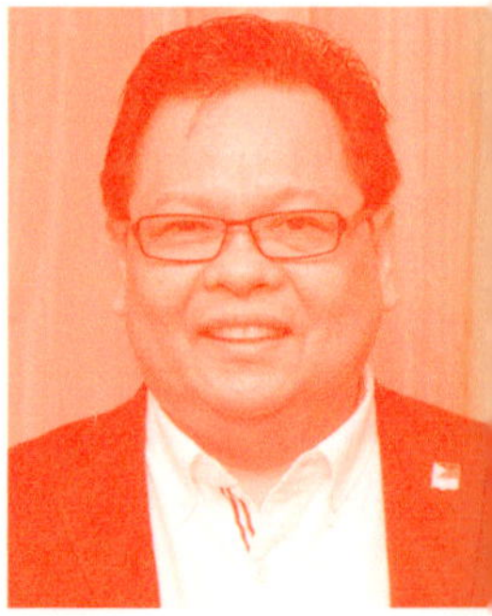
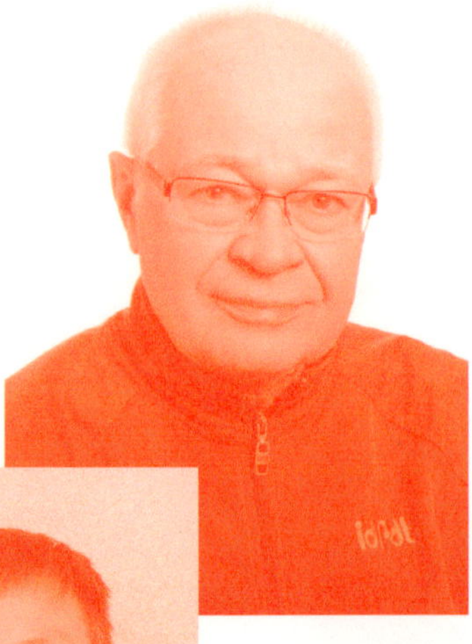
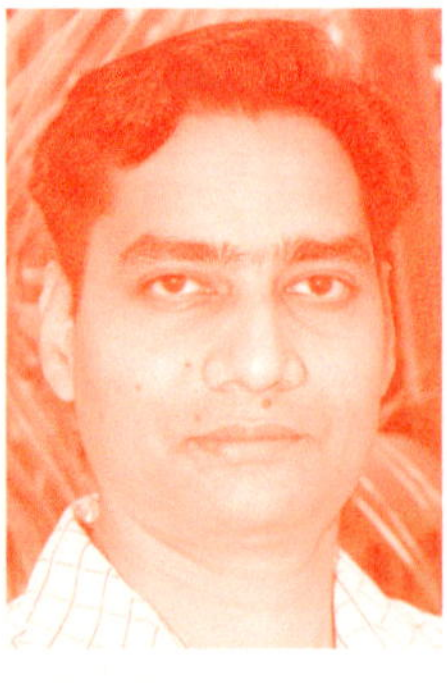
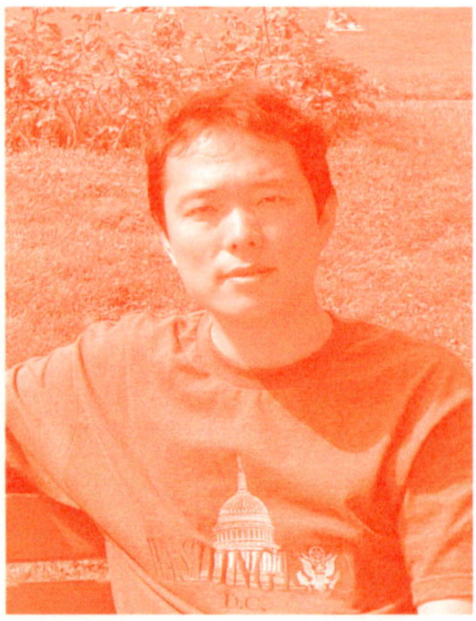
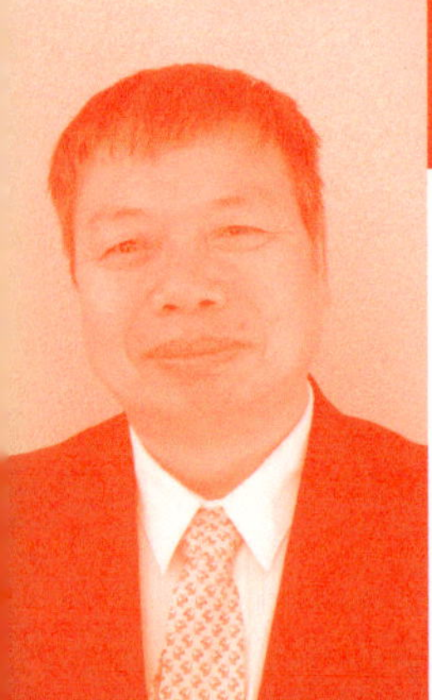
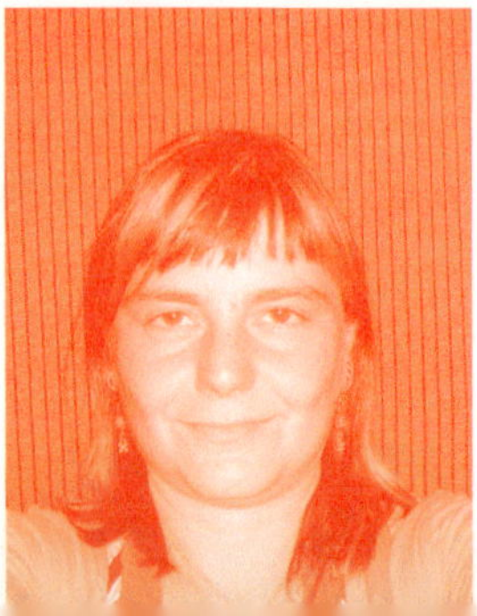

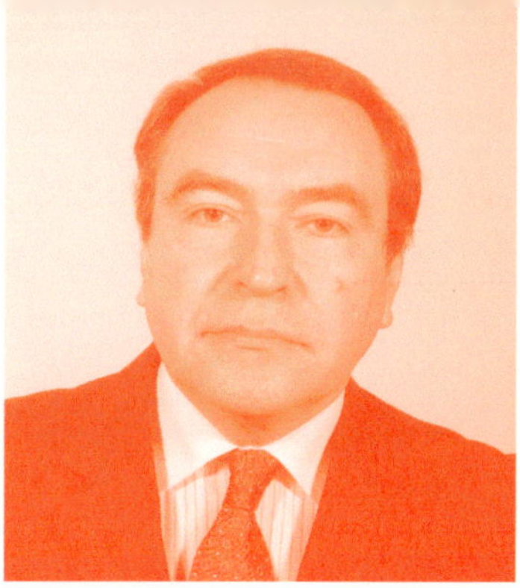
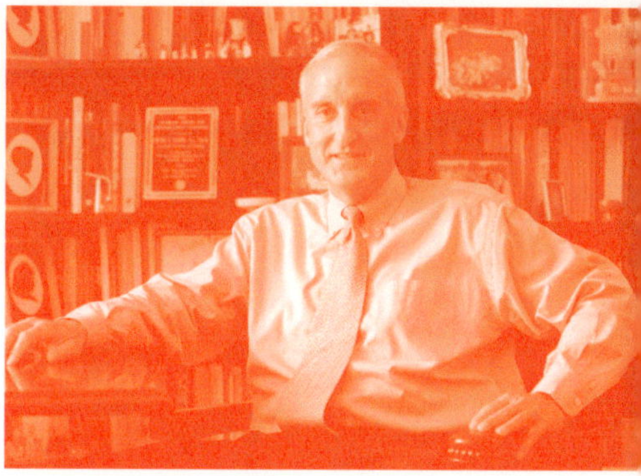
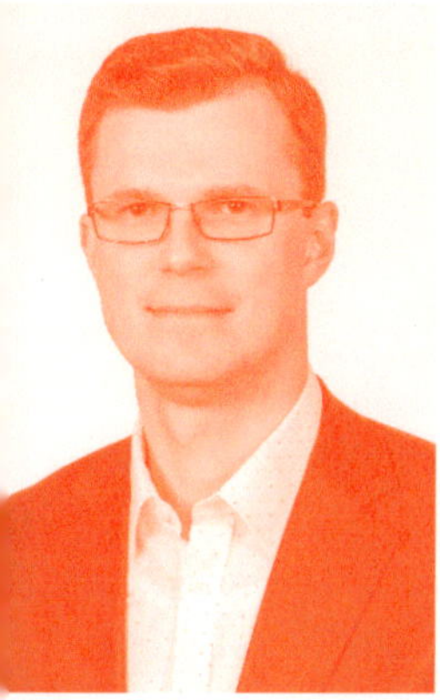
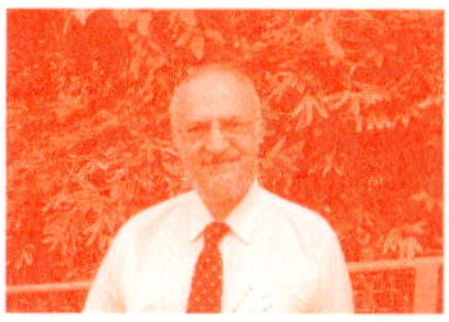
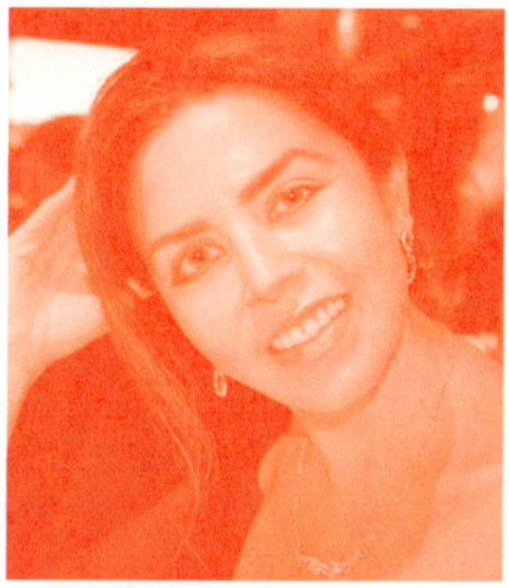

*Supporting open minds since 2005*

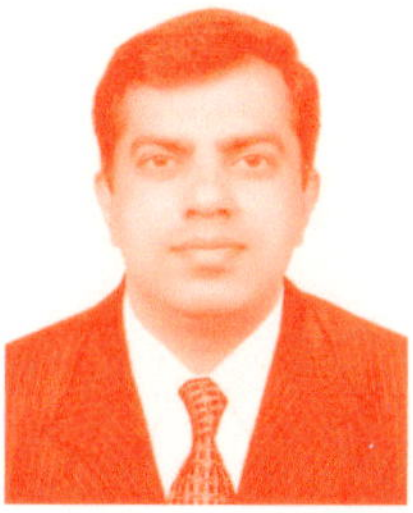
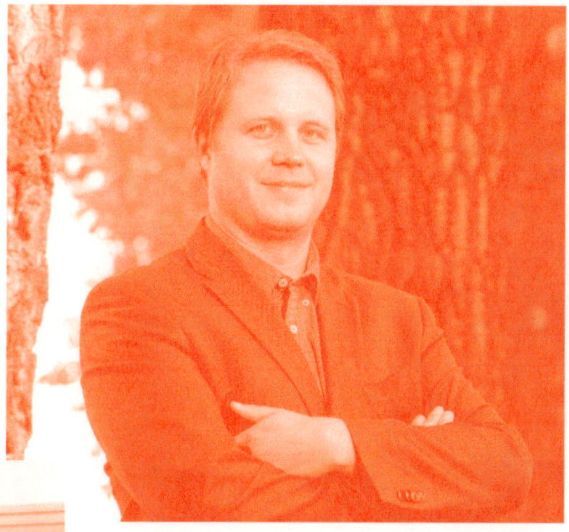
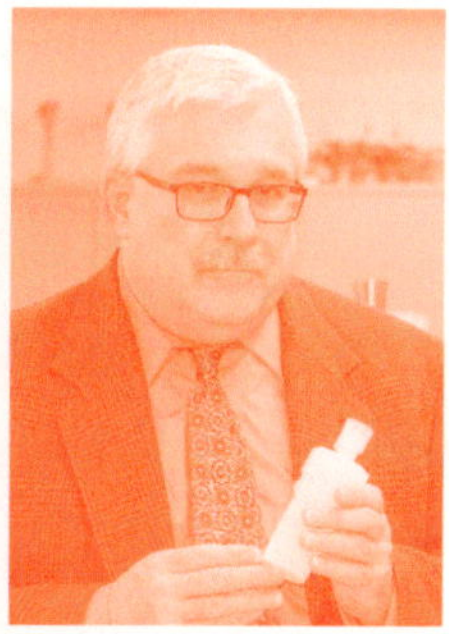
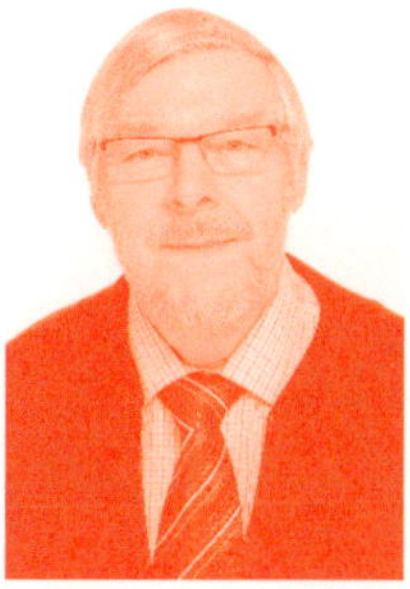
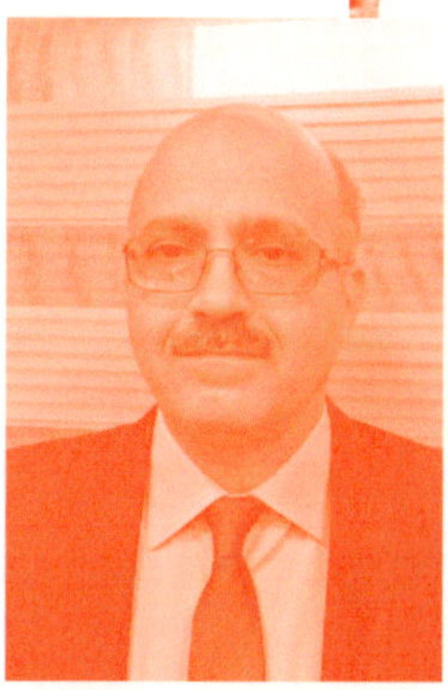
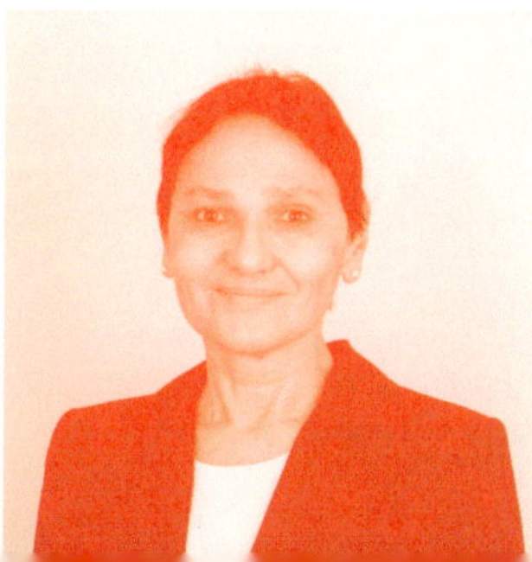
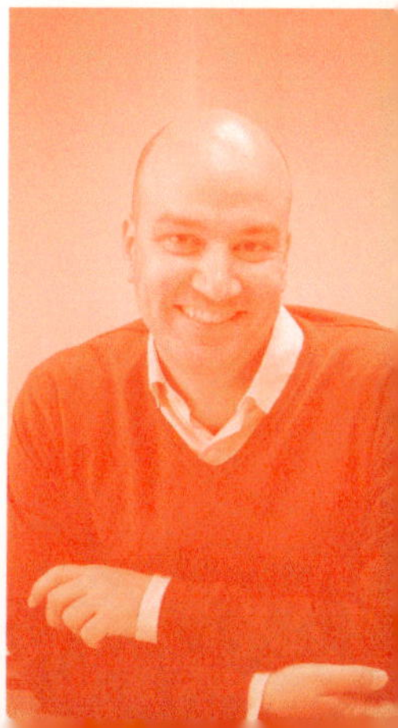

Snake Venom and Ecology
http://dx.doi.org/10.5772/intechopen.95194
Edited by Mohammad Manjur Shah, Umar Sharif, Tijjani Rufai Buhari and Tijjani Sabiu Imam

Contributors
Asirwatham Pushpa Arokia Rani, Marie Serena McConnell, Jeffrey D. Camper, Maniram Banjade, Hong-Shik Oh, Mamdouh Ibrahim Nassar, Mohammad Manjur Shah, Tijjani Sabiu Imam, Zainab Tukur, Aisha Bala



First published in London, United Kingdom, 2022 by IntechOpen
IntechOpen is the global imprint of INTECHOPEN LIMITED, registered in England and Wales, registration number: 11086078, 5 Princes Gate Court, London, SW7 2QJ, United Kingdom
Printed in Croatia

British Library Cataloguing-in-Publication Data
A catalogue record for this book is available from the British Library

Additional hard and PDF copies can be obtained from orders@intechopen.com

Snake Venom and Ecology
Edited by Mohammad Manjur Shah, Umar Sharif, Tijjani Rufai Buhari and Tijjani Sabiu Imam
p. cm.
Print ISBN 978-1-80355-063-3
Online ISBN 978-1-80355-064-0
eBook (PDF) ISBN 978-1-80355-065-7

For EU product safety concerns:
IN TECH d.o.o., Prolaz Marije Krucifikse Kozulić 3, 51000 Rijeka, Croatia, info@intechopen.com or visit our website at intechopen.com.

# Meet the editors

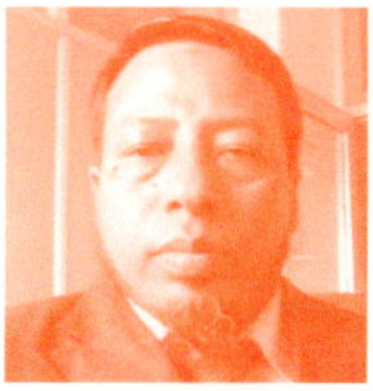

Dr. Mohammad Manjur Shah obtained a Ph.D. from Aligarh Muslim University (AMU), India, in 2003. He is a pioneer in the field of insect parasitic nematodes and has presented his findings at several conferences and published articles in various international journals. He completed two post-doctoral fellowships under the Ministry of Science and Technology, Government of India, before joining Yusuf Maitama Sule University Kano (YUMSUK), Nigeria, as an associate professor in 2015. Dr. Shah is the editor of six books and a reviewer for several scientific journals.

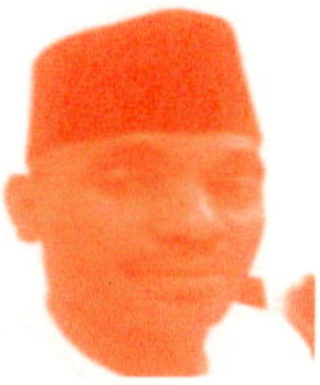

Dr. Umar Sharif obtained an MSc and Ph.D. from Bayero University Kano (BUK), Nigeria. Since 1990, he has been actively involved in teaching as well as various research programmes. He has good experience in the field of pathology. He is a member of various scientific societies in Nigeria and well versed in various fields of biology with constructive criticism and review. He has presented his findings at various conferences and published papers in journals of international repute.

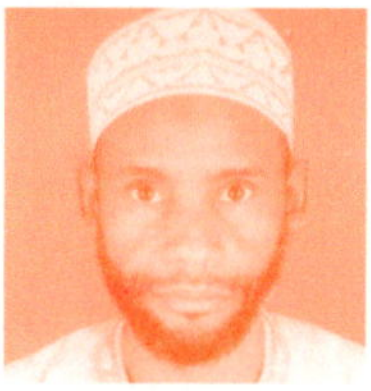

Dr. Tijjani Rufai Buhari obtained a Ph.D. from Universiti Putra Malaysia in 2012. At present, he is the director of Academic Planning, at Yusuf Maitama Sule University Kano (YUMSUK), Nigeria. Since 2007, he has been engaged in teaching and research in biology, particularly namely developmental biology, embryology, fisheries and aquaculture, marine biology, environmental microbiology, genetics, general biology, food and nutrition, and food sanitation. Apart from publishing many papers in journals of international repute, Dr. Buhari has attended and presented papers at many conferences, seminars, and workshops.

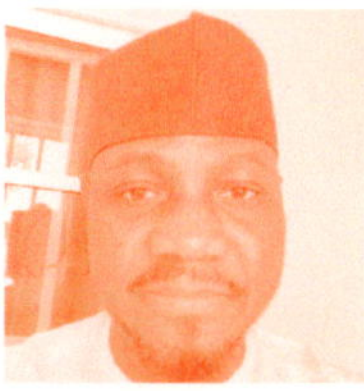

Dr. Tijjani Sabiu Imam obtained a Ph.D. in Environmental Biology from Bayero University Kano (BUK), Nigeria, in 2013. Currently, he is the head of the Department of Biology, BUK. He has been actively involved in teaching and research in addition to his various administrative responsibilities. He has published his findings in numerous international and national journals as well as in proceedings of scientific conferences, seminars, congregations, and workshops. His main areas of research are environmental biology, parasitology, and public health.

# Contents


**Preface** XI

**Section 1**
Toxins in Snake Venom 1

**Chapter 1** 3
Snake Venom
*by Asirwatham Pushpa Arokia Rani and Marie Serena McConnell*

**Chapter 2** 27
Snake Venom and Therapeutic Potential
*by Mamdouh Ibrahim Nassar*

**Chapter 3** 47
Survey of Snakes Bites among Snake Endemic Communities
in North Eastern Nigeria
*by Mohammad Manjur Shah, Tijjani Sabiu Imam, Aisha Bala
and Zainab Tukur*

**Section 2**
Snake Ecology 61

**Chapter 4** 63
Ecology of Red-Tongue Viper (*Gloydius ussuriensis*) in Jeju Island,
South Korea
*by Hong-Shik Oh and Maniram Banjade*

**Chapter 5** 77
Comparative Ecology of Two Species of Semiaquatic Snakes
in Southeastern North America
*by Jeffrey D. Camper*

# Preface

Snakes play a very important role in our ecosystem. They help in balancing the food web, regulating the population of their prey, and thereby controlling pests. They also exhibit both predator and prey characteristics and help in maintaining biodiversity on Earth for future sustainable development. This book highlights the extreme ecological importance of snakes with chapters on snake venom and its therapeutic potential and the ecology of some selected snake species.

**Dr. Mohammad Manjur Shah**
Department of Biological Sciences,
Yusuf Maitama Sule University,
Kano, Nigeria

**Dr. Umar Sharif and Dr. Tijjani Rufai Buhari**
Yusuf Maitama Sule University,
Kano, Nigeria

**Dr. Tijjani Sabiu Imam**
Byero University,
Kano, Nigeria

## Section 1

# Toxins in Snake Venom

Chapter 1

# Snake Venom

*Asirwatham Pushpa Arokia Rani*
*and Marie Serena McConnell*

## Abstract

Venomous snakes belonging to the family Viperidae, Elapidae, Colubridae and Hydrophidae, produces snake venom in order to facilitate immobilization and digestion of prey, act as defense mechanism against threats. Venom contains zootoxins which is a highly modified saliva that is either injected *via* fangs during a bite or spitted. The modified parotid gland, encapsulated in a muscular sheath, present on each side of the head, below and behind the eye, have large alveoli which temporarily stores the secreted venom and later conveyed by a duct to tubular fangs through which venom is injected. Venoms are complex mixtures of more than 20 different compounds, mostly proteins and polypeptides, including proteins, enzymes and substances with lethal toxicity which are either neurotoxic or haemotoxic in action and exert effects on nervous/muscular impulses and blood components. Lots of research are directed to use venoms as important pharmacological molecules for treating various diseases like Alzheimer's disease, Parkinson's disease etc.

**Keywords:** snake, venom, toxin, proteins, haemotoxic, neurotoxic, pharmacological molecules

## 1. Introduction

Snakes produce venoms that finds its use in immobilizing and digesting the prey and acts as an effective defense system against threats. Thus, venom is a functional trait utilized by an organism to regulate homeostatic processes of another organism i.e., it mediates the outcome of interactions between two or more organisms [1]. These snake venoms are storehouse of fascinating and useful bioactive compounds. Although various studies have been carried out on venoms, only few of them are well understood and tapped for their potential use in medicine as pharmacological molecules and diagnostics, understanding the molecular mechanisms of bodily processes such as homeostasis, coagulation, thrombosis, angiogenesis, and metastasis. The enthusiasm to understand animal envenomation and associated medical treatments has driven the animal venom studies in a multifaceted manner [2]. This chapter deals with what is venom, need for venom, evolution of venom, the poison apparatus that aids in producing the venom, genetics and biochemistry of the venom, effects of venom, antivenom, and applications of venom as therapeutics, diagnostics, and as biochemical tool.

## 2. Venom

Venom in layman's terms is modified snake saliva. This concoction is a combination of zootoxins, enzymes, and pharmacologically active peptides [3–5].

Digestive enzymes and other proteins that act as a paralyzing and pre-digestive agent. Digestion is therefore initiated outside the predator's alimentary canal while simultaneously immobilizing the prey. The snake then swallows the prey whole, liquefying most of the tissue and discarding what cannot be digested (feathers/hair/claws) along with the fecal matter. Although venomous snakes apply venom in the acquisition of the prey, they also fan out them in defensive bites against intimidating predators and aggressors.

## 2.1 The need for venom

Snakes are carnivores and actively hunt their prey. Most of them are ambush hunters and generalized feeders. Their geographic distribution and dietary preferences being varied, snakes had to evolve a method of incapacitating their prey quickly and their answer was venom. Geographic location and varied diet have led to the development of more and more complex venom. Being generalized feeders, many species of snake have a larger repertoire of proteins in their venom that affect individual prey animal species differently [6]. Honing the composition, mechanism of delivery, dosage and action of venom remains one of nature's greater success stories to date. Venom production has aided the proliferation and diversification of snakes as a group.

## 2.2 Evolution of venom in snakes

The evolution of snakes remains a partially solved mystery to scientists. Though they have known that snakes are descended from lizards since the 1970's there are many missing links due to a lack of proper fossil evidence. Debates of their descent from aquatic or terrestrial lizards persist as there is evidence to support both hypotheses. But the evolution of venom on the other hand has started to unravel. Initial research suggested that the venom and the venom delivery apparatus evolved together. But in 2002 a group of scientists in Australia led by Dr. B. Fry made amazing roads into the history of the evolution of venom. The major factor in the previous theory was that though many species had fangs they were in different locations in the jaw, size, and structure. The venom gland on the other hand remained the same.

Dr. Fry and his team examined the idea that the production of venom must predate the use of fangs. They looked at the extant lizard species which were said to contain toxins in their saliva. They discovered that the Komodo dragon and many of their related monitor lizards all had venom glands at the base of the lower jaw. This venom mixed with saliva caused damage to the prey previously thought to be caused by bacteria mixed in the saliva. The venom was like snake venom [7]. Most lizard species have been shown to have a gland like the venom gland of snakes, this led to the theory that snakes and lizards had a common venomous ancestor and that venom predated fangs.

Discoveries have shown around 1500 species of lizards had components like snake venom. Sea snakes are considered to have diverged from terrestrial snakes around 30 mya. Their venom is highly toxic. Studies have shown that they are evolving more complex toxin molecules to suit their ever-changing prey. This goes to show that venom is still evolving. The dietary preferences of the snake can magnify the change in venom. The snake can produce a potent mixture that can affect different prey animals uniquely [6]. There is no efficient antivenin generated against sea snakes.

There are so many species of snakes whose venom composition is yet to be studied in detail. These studies are crucial in understanding the evolution of venom and the effect of venom on prey species [8].

## 3. Poison apparatus

In reptiles, twice the venom glands have evolved; once in helodermatid lizards and secondly in advanced snakes belonging to colubroids, viperids, elapids and astractaspidids [9]. Venomous snakes belong to 4 genera. These snakes possess a poison apparatus or venom producing glands in their heads, which produces toxic substance that acts as either a poison or a venom. When the toxic substance is injected into the body of prey, it is venomous.

### 3.1 General plan

A poison apparatus of a snake consists of snakes consists of 4 major parts, namely, a pair of poison gland, poison ducts, fangs and muscles.

#### *3.1.1 Poison glands*

These glands situated on either side of the upper jaw, is possibly the superior labial glands or parotid glands. Each poison gland has a sac-like capsule and a narrow duct at the anterior end. The vascular fibrous septum of the capsule separates glandular substances into secretory pockets. The duct after passing along the sides of the upper jaw, opens at the base of the fang or at the base of the tunnel on the fang. The poison glands are held in position via anterior and posterior ligaments, which attaches anterior end of glands to maxilla and posterior end to the quadrate respectively. The fan shapes ligaments are situated between the side walls and squamosal-quadrate junction.

#### *3.1.2 Ducts*

The pair of ducts opens into a pocket of mucous sheath that covers the basal part of the fang. In spitting cobras (*Naja nigricollis*), the poison duct is modified into 'L' shaped bend prior to exiting the fang.

#### *3.1.3 Fangs*

The fangs evolved to inject venom into the prey is a grooved or tubular tooth. The paired pointed and hook-like teeth are modified form of maxillary teeth. They are long, curved, sharp and pointed. Based on the structure and position, fangs are of 3 types:

i. Proteroglyphous (Protero – first)
These are small, grooved, articulated at permanently erect at the anterior end of maxillae. They are found in Cobras, Kraits, Coral snakes and Sea snakes.

ii. Opisthoglyphous (Opistho - behind)
They are small and grooved but remain associated with posterior end of maxillae.

iii. Solenoglyphous (Solen – pipe; glyph - hollow)
This type of fangs is seen in vipers and rattle snakes. A large functional fang occurs on the front of each maxilla and are movable and turned inside to lie in the roof of mouth when it is closed. This fang contains a narrow hollow poison canal with enamel, which opens at anterior end of the fang.

### *3.1.4 Muscles*

Positioning and functioning of the poisonous apparatus is enabled by the presence of 3 types of muscle bands, namely, Digastrics, Sphenopterygoid, and Anterior and posterior temporalis.

## 3.2 Venom glands of elapidae

Early description about the elapid venom gland dates to 1936 [10]. *Elapidae* venom gland is enclosed in a tough capsule of connective tissue and more compactly built than that of viperid snakes. It consists of a posterior main gland and an anterior secretory duct with an accessory mucous gland. Simple or compound multiple contiguous tubules that run in a posterior–anterior direction is seen in the main gland. The tubules converge toward the centre of the gland and open into a small lumen. The secretory epithelium is of a serous nature. Secretory cells of elapids at resting stage are loaded with granules that differ in structure and number than those found in viperid venom gland. The cells of the accessory glands are PAS-positive, and their secretions mainly consists of sialomucins [11].

## 3.3 Venom glands of viperidae

The venom glands belonging to two viperid subfamilies, namely *Viperinae* and *Crotalinae* exhibit similarity in shape and structure. Except for the mole vipers belonging to the genus *Atractaspis*, all other have a glandular structure. The mole vipers differ in not possessing a differentiated accessory glands unique to the "genuine" vipers. The glands consist of large numbers of radial tubules surrounding a central lumen. The tubules are unbranched, and the luminal end consists of a mucous epithelium [12]. The venom of *Atractaspis engaddensis* has a relatively high alkaline monophaosphatase activity and is devoid of arginine ester hydrolase activity that is seen in other vipers. The first person to give a detailed account of venom glands of a true viper, *Vipera berus,* is Wolter in 1924 [13].

The venom gland has four distinct regions: the main gland, the primary duct, the accessory glands, and the secondary duct that leads to the fang sheath. The accessory glands have two distinct regions. The anterior part is lined by mucous epithelium that contains goblet cells while the posterior part is lined with flat to cuboidal epithelium, correlating with the secretory function [14]. The main gland is made of repeatedly branched tubules arranged around a large central lumen, where a considerable amount of venom can be stored. The tubules are made of secretory cells.

## 3.4 Venom glands of colubroidea

A pair of homologous oral venom glands located behind the eye on either side of the upper jaw are connected to the ducts that transfers the secreted venom to the base if morphologically diverse teeth, fangs [15].

## 3.5 Venom glands of sea snakes

The venom glands and related muscles of sea snakes are like the general structure that we observe in the terrestrial elapids. The considerable reduction in venom gland as well as the accessory gland is attributed to the aquatic environment. An early divergence of sea snakes from an ancestral elapis stock has been proposed as the musculus compressor glandulae is well developed in the sea snakes. A possible phylogenetic relationship exists between Australian elapids and hydrophiine snakes which is evident from the similarities that exists between them [16].

### 3.6 Changes in venom gland following milking process

Morphological changes in the secretory epithelium of venom gland after the expulsion of venom was noticed by Velikii in *Vipera ammodytes* [17] which was later confirmed by further studies [18, 19].

## 4. Genetics of snake venom

The bioactivity of the venom is determined by the complex and variable interactions between genes, their expression, their translation, and their post translational modification. Evidence that the loss of genes also has a strong influence on shaping venom phenotypes further reinforces the usage of animal venom systems to understand adaptation in the natural world is evident from the loss of genes that have a strong effect on forming the venom phenotype [20].

## 5. Biochemistry and physiology of snake venom

Venom was identified to be a proteinaceous concoction in the 1800s. 90 to 95% of the dry weight of venom is made of proteins. These proteins are also responsible for the biological effects of the venom. These proteins can be classified as enzymes and toxins [21]. The components of venom can vary from animal to animal within a species too. Research has shown that age [22], gender [23], geographic location [24], prey species/diet [25] and season [26] can all influence the composition of venom. All the proteins involved in venom are repurposed from regular physiological functions.

The proteins identified in venom have been studied individually, as protein complexes and as protein families. The proteins in the complex can be homodimers (made up of identical subunits) or heterodimers (made up of different subunits – sometimes these subunits are from different families). These complexes are held together by covalent bonds and the complexes are pharmacologically more potent than the individual enzymes or proteins. The complexes seem to expose critical residues that otherwise may have been buried in the individual enzymes [27].

### 5.1 Enzymes in snake venom

Typically, snake venom contains hundreds of components, all of which work in tandem to paralyze the prey and initiate digestion. Many enzymes are found and even some toxins have enzymatic functions. The most studied enzymes and their role are discussed below.

#### *5.1.1 5' Nucleotidase (5'-NT)*

This is an enzyme made up of 548 amino acids and a molecular mass of 61 kDa found in almost all living cells. The enzyme hydrolyses nucleosides. It is found in all snake venom around the world. Isoforms have also been isolated, like the isoform from the venom of *Vipera lebetina* (Cypriot blunt-nosed viper) that is found to be a homodimeric monomer with a molecular mass of 60 kDa. This isomer inhibits ADP- or Collagen-induced platelet aggregation [28]. The isomer isolated from the

Japanese pit viper (*Gloydius blomhoffii blomhoffii*) shows that the enzyme has 2 binding sites for Zn + and can exist as a trimer or a tetramer [29]. Venomous snakes belonging to the family Viperidae (*Vipera russelli russelli*- Russell's viper, *Echis carinatus*- Indian saw-scaled viper, *Eristocophis macmahonii* - Asian sand viper) were studied in the country of Pakistan and were all found to have high 5'-NT activity venom wise [30]. Among the snakes in Brazil that were studied, *Bothrops brazili* (Brazil's lancehead) had the highest 5'-NT activity. On the other hand, venom from *Philodryas olferssi* (South American green racer), a snake endemic to South America, showed little or no activity of 5'-NT. Among all the snakes studied there were differences in zymology and banding patterns among the enzymes thereby implying important physical structural differences [31]. The enzyme 5'-NT is found to act synergistically with other enzymes and have a pronounced anti-coagulant effect. It is said to liberate adenosine, and this helps immobilize the prey. In 2008, it was showed that the whole enzyme or a part of it is secreted in the venom. The soluble form of the enzyme is released by cleavage of the ectodomain in the venom gland or specialized tissues [29].

### *5.1.2 Acetylcholinesterase (AChE)*

It is the primary enzyme that catalyzes the breakdown of Acetylcholine in the body among other related neurotransmitters. AChE is found in nerve and muscle tissue, especially abundant in synaptic junctions. This is perhaps one of the well-studied enzymes from snake venom, its structure has been elucidated in detail. AChE is abundant in the venom of all snakes and higher concentrations are observed in the Elapid snakes except the Mambas [32]. Although the enzyme is present in the venom of snakes belonging to Viperidae and Crotalidae the activity was not detected. The highest concentration of venom AChE (VAChE) is found in the venom of *Bungarus* sp. 8 mg/gm of dried weight [33]. VAChE is found to be optimally active at 45° C and pH 8.5 [34].

The protein structure of VAChE shows homology to mammalian and Torpedo AChE with a few major changes. These changes ensure that VAChE has a less complicated structure than membrane-bound AChE. Many isoenzymes exist and can be differentiated on charge alone [35]. Protein structure has been studied from the VAChE of *Bungarus fasciatus* (BfAChE) and *Naja naja oxiana* (NnAChE). BfAChE exists as a soluble hydrophobic monomer. The C terminal peptide has an alternative exon ('S'). It is made up of 15 residues, the last 8 of these are removed in the mature protein. Compared to mammalian AChE, BfAChE has the following changes: Tyr70 is replaced by Met70, Acidic residue285 (glutamate/aspartate) is replaced by Lys285. The active site gorge is 20 A° deep and has two ligand-binding sites [36]. The crystallized structure shows evidence for a co-existing open/closed state in the back door channel and semi occuled gorge entrance. The presence of Met70 enlarges the entrance of the gorge, enabling better binding. It can form canonical dimers of subunits despite non-amphiphilic C terminus.

The NnAChE exists as a monomer at 0.2 mg/ml and a dimer at 2 mg/ml. It is a single polypeptide chain with a molecular weight of 67,000 ± 2000 Da and exists in several isoforms with different isoelectric points [37]. It differs from BfAChE by having a dimerization domain where His replaces Pro at position 514 [38]. VAChE has been associated with acute neuromuscular paralysis and neuromuscular weakness. This may be due to a defective transmission in the neuromuscular junction [5]. The function of AChE in elapid venoms could be to aid in the immediate hydrolysis of acetylcholine released from synaptic vesicles. This release could be under the influence of β-neurotoxin to avoid competitive protection by acetylcholine of postjunctional receptors against α-neurotoxin [39].

#### *5.1.3 Phosphatases–acid phosphatase (ACP) and alkaline phosphatase (ALP)*

These enzymes are found in lysosomes and during digestion they work on releasing the phosphoryl groups from molecules. They are found in all snake venoms. Both enzymes have a greater action in Elapids than Viperids. In a study that compared *Cerastes cerastes* (Saharan horned viper), *Cerestes vipers* (Saharan sand viper), *Naja haje* (Egyptian cobra) and *N. nigricollis* (Blacked neck spitting cobra) showed that *N. nagiricollis* showed higher ACP activity than ALP. But both enzymes needed $Mg^{++}$ to activate them [40]. The enzymes play an important role in liberating the purines, mainly Adenosine, thereby aiding immobilization of the prey organism. The Purines act as multi-toxins inducing hypotension and paralysis [41] *via* purine receptors in the prey's body [42].

#### *5.1.4 Hyaluronidase (Hyl)*

Hyaluronidases are a group of enzymes that are responsible for the degradation of Hyaluronic acid (HA), a glycosaminoglycan commonly found in abundance in nervous, epithelial, and connective tissues in all animals. Isolation and biological characterization of Hyl has been done from the venom of many snakes including *N. naja* – Indian Cobra [43], *Agkistrodon contortrix contortrix* – Eastern Copperhead [44], *C. cerastes* – Saharan Horned Viper [45], *Crotalus durissus terrificus* – South American Rattlesnake [46], *Bothrops pauloensis-* South American Pit viper and *Bungarus caerulecs* - Indian Krait. The snake Hyaluronidase (SHyl) from the venom of *Bungarus caerulecs* (Indian Krait) was found to have a molecular weight of 14 ± 2 kDa. The enzyme has an optimum temperature of 37°C and an optimum pH of 6 [47].

The cDNA of SHyl isolated *B. pauloensis* venom gland shows a protein with 194 amino acids synthesized from 1175 bps. The cDNA variants of SHyl isolated *Echis pyramidum leakeyi* (Kenyan Carpet Viper), *Echis carinatus sochureki* (Sochurek's saw-scaled viper) and *Bitis arietans* (Puff Adder) all show the presence of a truncated protein: Hy-L- 1000 that encodes the consensus amino- and carboxyl-termini with a central deletion of 256 residues, Hy-L-750 that lacks the consensus amino-terminus and Hy-L-500 that lacks the amino-terminus and encodes a shorter carboxy-terminal segment [48]. The SHyl is referred to as a 'Spreading factor' as it destroys the extracellular matrix (ECM). By degrading Hyaluronic acid, the enzyme increases the permeability of the tissue paving the way for the other venom toxins to act [49]. Many Hyaluronidase-type proteins have been identified in snake venom. These variants are produced by alternative splicing pathways. The Hyaluronidase-type proteins have not been isolated or characterized as they are highly temperature and pH-sensitive.

#### *5.1.5 Phospholipases*

These are enzymes that generally hydrolyze phospholipids into fatty acids and lipophilic substances. There are four major classes named A, B, C and D which are differentiated by the type of reaction they catalyze. Phospholipase A2 (PLA2) is found to be present in the venom of snakes and bees [50]. The enzyme acts on intact lectin molecules and hydrolyses the fatty acids esterified to the second carbon atom [51]. The venom enzymes are like mammalian enzymes in structure and function. The Phospholipase A2 enzymes found in venom are further grouped as I, II and IIE. Group I are major components of Elapidae venom, Group II are major components Viperidae venom [52] and IIE have been identified in the venom of non-front fanged snakes [53]. This enzyme which has a high affinity to specific receptors and a separate pharmacological site can target a large spectrum of tissues and thereby induce pharmacological effects which are dependent or independent of the catalytic activity of the enzyme.

There exist many unique examples of modulation of PLA2 activity generated by molecular evolution. The enzyme can exist as a homodimer, a post synaptic complex called Vipoxin (South-Eastern European Viper, *Vipera ammodytes meridionalis*). It is composed of PLA2 along with an acidic/catalytic inactive PLA2 like component called the inhibitor (Inh). Both components have 62% sequence homology. It is thought that the Inh acts to stabilize the enzyme component. It could have evolved from the catalytic molecule to the inhibitor [54]. Further studies have shown that a single change in amino acid sequence alters the function of the molecule. Gln48 PL A2 (*V. ammodytes meridionalis*) acts as a chaperone molecule and directs a toxic His48 PLA2 onto an acceptor. Homodimer of Gln48 PLA2 or His48 PLA2 is less toxic when compared to the heterodimer containing both Gln48 PLA2 and His48 PLA2. In another example, neonates of the Mexican jumping viper, *Metapilcoatlus* sp., have been reported to lack PLA2s but in contrast the adults have large quantities of the enzyme. But the venom of both the neonates and the adults was found to be haemorrhagic [55].

### *5.1.6 L-amino acid oxidases*

L-amino acid oxidases (LAAOs) are multifunctional enzymes. They produce hydrogen peroxide and ammonia as part of their catalytic activity. These are highly toxic and can destroy major components of the cell viz. nucleic acids, proteins and the plasma membrane [56]. Snake venom L-amino acid oxidases (SVLAAOs) were first detected in the venom of *Vipera aspis*. SVLAAOs are homodimers with cofactors FAD (Flavin Adenine Dinucleotide) or FMD (Flavin Mononucleotide) linked covalently. Abundance of Riboflavin, also a pigment, is a major contributor to the yellow color of snake venom [57].

SVLAAOs vary between snake species. The enzymes when injected into the prey cause the formation of oxygen reactive species extracellularly. These highly toxic oxygen reactive species, hydrogen peroxide and ammonia, alter the permeability of the plasma membrane and induce apoptosis, which in turn leads to cell death [58]. The SVLAAOs are dependent on ions for activation and inactivation. The LAAOs found in the venom of *Crotalus adamanteus*, Eastern Diamondback rattlesnake, require $Mg^{2+}$ to be activated [59], whereas the enzymes in the venom of *Lachesis muta*, South American Bushmaster, and *Bothrops brazli*, Lancehead pit viper, are inhibited by the binding of $Zn^{2+}$ [60].

Analysis of the sequences of SVLAAOs from around the globe showed ~60% similarity. The most dissimilar regions were the C and N terminals of the protein. Most SVLAAOs are rich in asparagine, glutamic acid and aspartic acid residues. The number of cysteine residues varies implying variation in the tertiary structure of these proteins [61].

### *5.1.7 Metalloproteinases*

Metalloproteinases are typically enzymes that depend on a metal ion to aid their catalytic activity. Snake venom Metalloproteinases (SVMPs) are Zinc ($Zn^{2+}$) dependent enzymes. Their size ranges from 20 to 110 kDa. They are broadly grouped into three (PI, PII, PIII) based on their structural domains. SVMPs in their varied isoforms are responsible for heaemorrhagic and coagulopathic nature of snake venoms. The SVMPs act on the different stages of the blood clotting pathway [62, 63].

### 5.2 Toxins in snake venom

The myriad of toxins found in snake venom are biologically costly to produce but potent and snakes have invested years of evolution to refine them. Many other toxins are species-specific and have been grouped by their pharmacological action to enable easy study. Though many toxins have been named, the neurotoxins and hemotoxins dominate them all. The identification, isolation characterization and evolution of snake venom toxins have been an area of prolific research since the 1970s.

#### *5.2.1 Neurotoxins in snake venom: three-finger toxin (3FTx) super family*

Many of the toxins predominant in snake venom belong to the three-finger toxin (3FTx) family. The group is named for the specific protein fold of three β strand loops connected to a central core with four disulphide bonds. This is a conserved feature. The proteins in this family are at an average of 60 to 74 amino acid residues in length [64]. These 3FTxs are peculiar to snakes although the superfamily of three-fold proteins is common to all eukaryotes [65]. Studies have shown that the 3FTxs of snakes have evolved from non-toxic three-finger proteins [3].

The number of 3FTxs varies from species to species. Elapsid and Colubrid venom are found to be abundant in 3FTxs [66]. 95% of the proteins in the venom of *Micrurus tschudii*, the desert coral snake [67], 70% of the proteins in the venom of *Ophiophagus hannah*, the King Cobra [68] and *Dendroaspis angusticeps*, the Eastern green mamba [69] are 3FTxs. These toxins bind post-synaptically and induce flaccid paralysis in the prey animal.

The structural differences between members of the family are broadly based on the length and number of disulphide bridges. - the longer 3FTxs with a chain length of 66–74 residues with 5 disulphide bridges (Examples: α-neurotoxins, γ-neurotoxins, hannalgesin, κ-neurotoxins) and the shorter chains with a chain length of 57–62 residues with 4 disulphide bridges (Examples: α-neurotoxins, β-cardiotoxins, cytotoxins, fasciculins and mambalgins). The 3FTxs can exist as covalent/non-covalent homo or heterodimers.

The mechanism of action of 3FTxs is varied despite them all having the same 3-finger fold. α-neurotoxins have been shown to inhibit acetylcholine receptors in muscle synapses [70]. κ-neurotoxins on the other hand inhibit acetylcholine receptors in neural synapses [71], fasciculins inhibit acetylcholinesterase [72], mambin interacts with platelet receptors [73], mambaligins inhibit ASIC channels [74] and calliotoxin activates voltage-gated sodium channel [75] to name just a few. It is to be noted that no 3FTxs are involved in inflammation and hyperalgesia typical of other snake toxins. The 3Ftxs target many ion channels and receptors in the prey animal. This is attributed to the unique capacity of the 3-finger fold and its ability to modulate diverse biological functions. Specific amino acid sequences in critical segments of 3FTxs have been identified, these sequences play an important role in binding to the target sites. The interactions of Acetylcholinesterase in the prey with the 3 loops in the fasciculin molecule show the first look of the fasciculin interaction with the outer enzyme but the second loop is inserted in the active site with hydrogen bonding (Lys 25, Arg24, Asn47, Pro31, Leu35 and Ala12) and hydrophobic interactions (Lys32, Cys59, Val34, Leu48, Ser26, Gly36, Thr15 and Asn20) [76]. The interactions of Muscarinic toxins from mamba venom [77], Neurotoxin II (NTII) from the venom of *Naja oxiana*, the Central Asian Cobra [78], Neurotoxin b (NTb) from the venom of O. hannah, King Cobra [79] have all been studied in detail and reports show the importance of the amino acid sequence in binding and modifying the action of the receptors. Any change in these sequences leads to loss of neurotoxicity of the molecule.

#### *5.2.2 Cardiotoxins/cytotoxins*

These toxins attack the cardiac muscle preventing muscle contraction. This leads to the irregularity of heartbeat and ultimately stopping of the heart. Experiments have shown that the toxins tend to bind to the surface of the muscle and cause depolarization. These toxins are ample in mamba venom and few species of cobra venom. Other cardiotoxins interact non-specifically with phospholipids [80] or induce insulin secretion [81]. B – cardiotoxins inhibit β-adrenoreceptors [82].

Cardiotoxins are single chain, small molecular weight (~ 6.5 kDa) proteins that are highly basic (pI>10). They exhibit a broad spectrum of pharmacological action. The cardiotoxins share significant sequence homology to neurotoxins yet despite this homology they display remarkably different properties. As many as 52 cardiotoxins have been reported and they have a 90% homology of sequence among themselves [83]. Cardiotoxin III (CTx III, Cytotoxin 3) is a 60-residue long toxin peculiar to the Taiwan Cobra (*Naja atra*). It can induce apoptosis in cells via the release of cytochrome [84]. The structure of cardiotoxin VII4 isolated from *Naja mossambica mossambica*, the Mozambique spitting cobra, was crystalized proving it was a dimer and have a molecular mass of 6715 Da. Studies have shown the cardiotoxin blocked nicotinic acetylcholine receptors [85].

A set of proteins called Cardiotoxin-like basic proteins (CLBP) are found to have homology with cardiotoxins but where cardiotoxins have the triple peptide signature (-I-D-V-) between 39 and 41, CLBPs lack this. Other differences include CLBPs having a Gln at 17 which is absent in cardiotoxins. CLBPs also lack the Met residue needed for activity [86]. These molecules are now being assessed for therapeutic ability.

## 6. Effects of snake bite and snake venom

Snake bite is a neglected public health issue in many tropical and subtropical countries. According to WHO (2021), an annual record of about 5.4 million snake bites and 1.8 to 2.7 million cases of envenomings has been reported. They have also reported that about 140,000 deaths occur. Bites by venomous snakes can cause acute medical emergencies involving severe paralysis that may prevent breathing, cause bleeding disorders that can lead to fatal hemorrhage, cause irreversible kidney failure and severe local tissue destruction that can cause permanent disability and limb amputation. The more severe effects experienced by the children is because of their smaller body mass [87].

The response of neurotoxicity to snake antivenom is dependent on the type of neurotoxins that the snake possess. Cobra venom contains post-synaptic nerutoxins that produce curare-like effect and hence can be reversed by snake antivenom after clinical effects have developed. While krait venom which contains many pre-synaptic neurotoxins, causes paralysis that is irreversible once developed and hence their response to antivenom is very poor [88, 89].

## 7. Antivenom

One of the major public health issues in the rural tropics is snake bites. Currently, the only specific treatment available to ameliorate the effect of snake bite is antivenom [90]. Snake antivenom was produced by raising hyperimmune serum in animals, such as horses. The hyerimmune serum was further purified to produce whole immunoglobulin G (IgG) antivenoms and then fractionated to F(ab) and $F(ab')_2$ antivenoms to reduce adverse reactions and increase efficacy.

A significant challenge in manufacturing of antivenoms is the preparation of the correct immunogens (snake venoms). At present very few countries have capacity to produce snake venoms of adequate quality for antivenom manufacture, and many manufacturers rely on common commercial sources [87]. Poor data on the number and type of snake bites have led to difficulty in estimating needs, and deficient distribution policies have further contributed to manufacturers reducing or stopping production or increasing the prices of antivenoms. Weak regulation and the marketing of inappropriate or poor quality antivenoms has also resulted in a loss of confidence in some of the available antivenoms by clinicians, health managers, and patients, which has further eroded demand.

## 8. Applications of snake venoms

### 8.1 Therapeutic implications

Snake venom consists of pharmacologically active proteins and peptides. The snake venoms show a distinct complexity from other animal venoms in that they possess a diverse array of proteins and peptides with wide range of pharmacological and toxicological effects.

#### *8.1.1 Snake venom-based drugs*

Based on the pharmacological effects produced, snake venom has been classified into haemotoxic, neurotoxic and cytotoxic venom. Although snake venoms are considered as mini drug libraries, only about 0.01% venom has been characterized. Snake venom is considered a valuable source of new principal compounds in drug discovery. Components of snake venom such as PLA2, serine proteases, metalloproteinase, lectins, l-amino acid oxidases, bradykinin potentiating factors, natriuretic factors, integrin antagonists possess pharmacological properties and exhibit neurotoxicity, myotoxicity, cytotoxicity, hemotoxicity, antimicrobial activity, which in turn exerts its action and disrupts the central and peripheral nervous systems, the blood coagulation cascade, the cardiovascular and neuromuscular systems and the general homeostasis state [5].

Importance of snake venom in medicine dates to thousands of years in Ayurveda, homeopathy and traditional or folk medicines. Cobra venom is used in the ayurvedic treatment of joint pain, inflammation, and arthritis [91] and other body fluids such as blood and bile duct in Chinese medicine [92] and lots of the snake venom-based drugs are available in the market and in clinical trials [93].

Various drugs based on snake venom in the market are Captopril® (Enalapril), Integrilin® (Eptifibatide) and Aggrastat® (Tirofiban) and many more are in the pipeline at pre-clinical or clinical trial stage [94]. Captopril®, approved by FDA in 1981, was the first successful drug derived from snake venom [95]. This drug is a biomimetic of bradykinin-potentiating peptide, isolated from the venom of Brazilian arrowhead viper *Bothrops jararaca*, was discovered by the Nobel prize winner Sir John Vane and its commercial production was taken care of by the pharmaceutical giant Squibb. It finds its use in treating hypertension and cardiovascular disease, where it acts by inhibiting the angiotensin converting enzyme that converts angiotensin I to angiotensin II [96].

Two drugs based on snake venom disintegrins, Aggrastat® (Tirofiban) marketed by Medicure Pharma in the US and Correvio International outside US, and Integrilin® (Eptifibatide) developed by Millennium Pharmaceuticals and co-promoted by Schering-Plow (which are both now part of Merck and Takeda Pharmaceuticals) are used as antiplatelet agents [97]. Aggrastat, belonging to the platelet glycoprotein (GP) IIb/IIIa inhibitors and developed based on the RGD sequence (Arg-Gly-Asp) motif from snake venom disintegrins isolated from the venom of *E. carinatus* is administered to treat heart attack patients [98]. Integrilin, which is used for treating acute coronary syndrome, is a peptide drug which mimics a small portion of the glycoprotein (GP) IIb/IIIa inhibitor barbourin found in the venom of the Southeastern pygmy rattlesnake (*Sistrurus miliarus barbouri*) based on the KGD sequence (Lys-Gly-Asp) [99]. Both Aggrastat® and Integrilin® was approved for medical use by FDA in 1998.

Defibrase®/Reptilase® (Batroxobin), a drug based on the thrombin-like serine protease enzyme isolated from the snake venom of two subspecies *Bothrops atrox* and *Bothrops moojeni* [100] is an approved drug mainly used in China to treat a range of disorders, including stroke, pulmonary embolism, deep vein thrombosis, myocardial infarction and perioperative bleeding. Another drug derived from the venom of *B. atrox*, Hemocoagulase® has been widely used in plastic surgery, abdominal surgery, and human vitrectomy [101]. Exanta® (Ximelagatran) derived from cobra venom, a thrombin inhibitor anticoagulant, is used as blood thinner and thrombin inhibitor [102].

Botrocetin® is a drug that is developed based on the platelet aggregating protein from the venom of *B. jararaca* and it is found to enhance the affinity of the von Willebrand factor A1 domain for the platelet receptor glycoprotein Ibalpha (GPIbalpha) [103]. The thrombin like serine proteinase RVV-V from *Vipera husselli* venom, an activator of factor V of the blood coagulation cascade, is tried for destabilizing and selectively inactivating factor V in plasma [104]. Ecarin, a metalloprotease isolated from the venom of the saw-scaled viper (*E. carinatus*) is used as prothrombin activator [105].

### *8.1.2 Putative therapeutic substances*

Taipoxin, a powerful presynaptic neurotoxin from *Oxyuranus scutellatus* (Australian taipan) snake venom, consists of three polypeptides, referred as alpha, beta, and gamma subunits. Trypsin degradation of the β-subunit yields Oxynor which has pharmacological properties against wounds [106]. Oxynor was subjected to clinical development by Ophidia Products, Inc., but no further progress has reported in literature.

Vicrostatin (VCN) is a chimeric disintegrin, made by the fusion of echistatin and contortrostatin, seen in crotalids snake venom. When VCN, packaged in liposome (LVCN), was intravenously administered *in vivo* to breast cancer models, a delayed tumor growth and prolong animal survival was observed [107]. The drug was in pre-clinical studies by Applied Integrin Sciences Inc., but no further progress has reported in literature.

*In vitro* studies of Salmosin, a disintegrin of 7.8 kDa (73 residues), isolated from *Agkistrodon halys brevicaudus* (Korean mamushi) venom, demonstrated its capacity to inhibit the proliferation of bovine capillary endothelial cells, induced by bFGF (basic fibroblast growth factor) by competing with ECM for binding with $\alpha v\beta 3$, detaches cells, and inactivates FAK-dependent signaling pathways, thereby leading to apoptosis [108]. Hence, Salmosin could be used as an anticancer agent in future.

Hannalgesin, an α-neurotoxin of approximately 7.9 kDa (72 residues) isolated from *O. hannah* (King cobra) venom, exhibits analgestic effect through nitric oxide or opioid systems. Its analgesic effect is higher than morphine [109].

### 8.2 Diagnostics

The feature of not being not affected by therapeutic or physiological coagulation inhibitors [Marsh, 2002], it has been applied for the analysis of hemostatic parameters, such as fibrinogen (dysfibrinogenemia, its breakdown products), antithrombin III, prothrombin (dysprothrombinaemias), von Willebrand factor (vWF), blood clot- ting factors (V, VII, X), protein C (PC), activated protein C (APC), and lupus anticoagulants (LA) [110]. Protac® and Proc Global assay, reptilase® and reptilase time, Anti-nAChR antibodies assay, textarin time, botrocetin®, RVV-V, RVV-X, and dRVVT (dilute Russell's viper venom time), *etc.* are the tests available [111].

### 8.3 Biochemical tool

The structures, functions and molecular mechanisms of receptors/ ion-channels that exhibit high potency, selectivity, and efficacy can be studied using snake venom peptides as molecular probes [112]. α- neurotoxins such as erabutoxin, α-cobratoxin, and α- bungarotoxin have high affinity for nicotinic acetylcholine receptors (nAChR). This feature is applied in isolating the α-bungarotoxin, from *Bungarus* sp. [113]. The muscarinic neurotoxins (MTs) or mamba toxin produced by *D. angusticeps* (green mamba) and related species is composed of 64–66 amino acids, homologous to α-neurotoxins and are highly selective for muscarinic receptor subtypes (mAChRs) [114]. This study gains importance in studying the role of mAChRs in Alzheimer's disease using mamba toxin and used as therapeutic agent in treating Alzheimer's and Parkinson's disease as it selectively blocks the receptor sub-types [115]. Dendrotoxins and related proteins, from *Dendroaspis* species (mamba snakes), belonging to sub-family of voltage-dependent potassium channels, are homologous to Kunitz-type serine protease inhibitors, composed of 57–60 amino acids polypeptide chain that is stabilized by the presence of three disulphide bridges. Therefore, these toxins could serve as biochemical tools to study various sub-type of L-type calcium channels.

## 9. Conclusions

Snake venoms are complex mixtures of toxins that exhibit interspecies and intraspecies variation due to the rapidly evolving and diverging venom genes in relation to the geographical area, environmental niches etc. The efficacy of snake venom is influenced by these variations. Future implications on the venom study are in the direction for search of effective pharmacological and diagnostic products.

## Conflict of interest

"The authors declare no conflict of interest."

## Author details

Asirwatham Pushpa Arokia Rani* and Marie Serena McConnell
PG and Research Department of Zoology, Lady Doak College, Affiliated to Madurai Kamaraj University, Madurai, Tamil Nadu, India

*Address all correspondence to: aparani@ldc.edu.in

## References

[1] Jackson TNW, Jouanne H, Vidal N. Snake venom in context: Neglected clades and concepts. Frontiers in Ecology and Evolution. 2019;7:332. DOI: 10.3389/fevo.2019.00332

[2] Zhang Y. Why do we study animal toxins? Dongwuxue Yanjiu. **2015;36**(4): 183-222. DOI: 10.13918/j.issn.2095-8137. 2015.4.183

[3] Casewell NR, Wüster W, Vonk FJ, Harrison RA, Fry BG. Complex cocktails: The evolutionary novelty of venoms. Trends in Ecology & Evolution. 2013;**28**(4):219-229. DOI: 10.1016/j.tree.2012.10.020

[4] Chan YS, Cheung RCF, Xia LX, Wong JH, Ng TB, Chan WY. Snake venom toxins: Toxicity and medicinal applications. Applied Microbiology and Biotechnology. 2016;**100**(14):6165-6181. DOI: 10.1007/s00253-016-7610-9

[5] Ferraz Camila R, Arif A, Chunfang X, Casewell Nicholas R, Lewis Richard J, Kool J, et al. Multifunctional toxins in snake venoms and therapeutic implications: from pain to hemorrhage and necrosis. Frontiers in Ecology and Evolution. 2019;7:218. DOI: 10.3389/fevo.2019.00218

[6] Holding ML, Strickland JL, Rautsaw RM, Hofmann EP, Mason AJ, Hogan MP, et al. Phylogenetically diverse diets favor more complex venoms in North American pit vipers. Proceedings of the National Academy of Sciences of the United States of America. 2021;**118**(17):1-10. DOI: 10.1073/pnas.2015579118

[7] Fry BG, Vidal N, Norman JA, Vonk FJ, Scheib H, Ramjan SFR, et al. Early evolution of the venom system in lizards and snakes. Nature. 2006; **439**(7076):584-588. DOI: 10.1038/nature04328

[8] Damm M, Hempel BF, Süssmuth RD. Old World vipers—a review about snake venom proteomics of viperinae and their variations. Toxins. 2021;**13**(6):427. DOI: 10.3390/toxins13060427

[9] Kochva E. Oral glands of the Reptilia. In: Gans C, Gans KA, editors. Biology of the Reptilia. Vol. 8. New York: Academic Press; 1978. pp. 43-94

[10] Bobeau G. Histo-phisiologie normale et pathologique de la glande à venin du Cobra. Bulletin de la Société Royale des Sciences Médicales et Naturelles de Bruxelles. **36**:53-58

[11] Rosenberg HI. Histology, histochemistry, and emptying mechanism of the venom glands of some elapid snakes. Journal of Morphology. 1967;**123**(2):133-155. DOI: 10.1002/jmor.1051230204

[12] Kochva E, Shayer-Wollberg M, Sobol R. The special pattern of venom gland in *Atractaspis* and its bearing on the taxonomic status of the genus. Copeia. 1967;**1967**(4):763-772. DOI: 10.2307/1441887

[13] Wolter M. Die Giftdrüse von *Vipera berus* L. Jenaische Zeitschrift für Medicin und Naturwissenschaft. 1924;**60**:305-357

[14] Kochva E, Gans C. Histology and histochemistry of venom glands of some crotaline snakes. Copeia. 1966;**1966**(3):506-515. DOI: 10.2307/1441074

[15] Kochva E. The development of the venom gland in the opisthoglyph snake Telescopus fallax with remarks on Thamnophis sirtalis (Colubridae, Reptilia). Copeia. 1965;**1965**(2):147-154. DOI: 10.2307/1440716

[16] Gopalakrishnakone P, Kochva E. Venom glands and some associated

muscles in sea snakes. Journal of Morphology. 1990;**205**(1):85-96. DOI: 10.1002/jmor.1052050109, PMID 29865733

[17] Velikii VN. O nervnykh okonchaniyakh v zhelezakh yadovitykh zmei. Trudy S-Perterburgs-kogo Obshcheva estestvoispytatelei. Otdelenie Zool Fiziologgi. 1890;**21**:16-17

[18] Ben-Shaul Y, Lifshitz S, Kochva E. Ultrastructural aspects of secretion in the venom glands of *Vipera palaestinae*. In: Toxins of Animal and Plant Origin. Vol. I. London: Gordon & Breach; 1971. pp. 87-105

[19] Rotenberg D, Bamberger ES, Kochva E. Studies on ribonucleic acid synthesis in the venom glands of *Vipera palaestinae* (Ophidia, Reptilia). The Biochemical Journal. 1971;**121**(4):609-612. DOI: 10.1042/bj1210609

[20] Casewell NR. Venom evolution: gene loss shapes phenotypic adaptation. Current Biology Dispatch. 2016;**26**(18):PR849-PR851. DOI: 10.1016/j.cub.2016.07.082

[21] Ferraz Camila R, Arif A, Chunfang X, Casewell Nicholas R, Lewis Richard J, Kool J, et al. Multifunctional toxins in snake venoms and therapeutic implications: From pain to hemorrhage and necrosis. Frontiers in Ecology and Evolution. 2019;**7**:218. DOI: 10.3389/fevo.2019.00218

[22] Dias GS, Kitano ES, Pagotto AH, Sant'anna SS, Rocha MM, Zelanis A, et al. Individual variability in the venom proteome of juvenile Bothrops jararaca specimens. Journal of Proteome Research. 2013;**12**(10):4585-4598. DOI: 10.1021/pr4007393

[23] Zelanis A, Menezes MC, Kitano ES, Liberato T, Tashima AK, Pinto AF, et al. Proteomic identification of gender molecular markers in Bothrops jararaca venom. Journal of Proteomics. 2016;**139**:26-37. DOI: 10.1016/j.jprot.2016.02.030

[24] Gonçalves-Machado L, Pla D, Sanz L, Jorge RJB, Leitão-De-Araújo M, Alves MLM, et al. Combined venomics, venom gland transcriptomics, bioactivities, and antivenomics of two Bothrops jararaca populations from geographic isolated regions within the Brazilian Atlantic rainforest. Journal of Proteomics. 2016;**135**:73-89. DOI: 10.1016/j.jprot.2015.04.029

[25] Barlow A, Pook CE, Harrison RA, Wüster W. Coevolution of diet and prey-specific venom activity supports the role of selection in snake venom evolution. Proceedings of the Biological Sciences. 2009;**276**(1666):2443-2449. DOI: 10.1098/rspb.2009.0048

[26] Gubensek F, Sket D, Turk V, Lebez D. Fractionation of Vipera Ammodytes venom and seasonal variation of its composition. Toxicon. 1974;**12**(2):167-171. DOI: 10.1016/0041-0101(74)90241-4

[27] Doley R, Kini RM. Protein complexes in snake venom. Cellular and Molecular Life Sciences. 2009;**66**(17):2851-2871. DOI: 10.1007/s00018-009-0050-2

[28] Trummal K, Samel M, Aaspõllu A, Tõnismägi K, Titma T, Subbi J, et al. 5'-Nucleotidase from Vipera lebetina venom. Toxicon. 2015 January; **93**:155-163. DOI: 10.1016/j.toxicon.2014.11.234

[29] Ogawa Y, Kanai-Azuma M, Akimoto Y, Kawakami H, Yanoshita R. Exosome-like vesicles in Gloydius blomhoffii blomhoffii venom. Toxicon. 2008;**51**(6):984-993. ISSN 0041-0101. DOI: 10.1016/j.toxicon.2008.02.003

[30] Mahmood AJ. Rashida Qasim and Syed Mahmood Alam enzymatic activities of some snake venoms from families Elapidae and Viperidae

Pakistan. Journal of Pharmaceutical Sciences. 1996;**9**(1):37-41

[31] Sales PB, Santoro ML. LNucleotidase and DNase activities in Brazilian snake venoms. Comparative Biochemistry and Physiology, Part C: Toxicology & Pharmacology. 2008;**147**(1):85-95. ISSN 1532-0456. DOI: 10.1016/j.cbpc.2007.08.003

[32] Cousin X, Bon C. Acetylcholinesterase from snake venom as a model for its nerve and muscle counterpart. Journal of Natural Toxins. 1999;**8**(2):285-294

[33] Frobert Y, Créminon C, Cousin X, Rémy MH, Chatel JM, Bon S, et al. Acetylcholinesterases from Elapidae snake venoms: biochemical, immunological and enzymatic characterization. Biochimica et Biophysica Acta. 1997;**1339**(2):253-267. DOI: 10.1016/s0167-4838(97)00009-5

[34] Ahmed M, Latif N, Khan RA, Ahmad A, Rocha JBT, Mazzanti CM, et al. Enzymatic and biochemical characterization of Bungarus sindanus snake venom acetylcholinesterase. Journal of Venomous Animals and Toxins Including Tropical Diseases. 2012;**18**(2):236-243. ISSN 1678-9199. DOI: 10.1590/S1678-91992012000200014

[35] Lee S-R, Latta J, Elliott LL. Comparative Biochemistry & Physiology. 1977;**56C**:193-197

[36] Rosenberry TL, Johnson JL, Cusack B, Thomas JL, Emani S, Venkatasubban KS. Interactions between the peripheral site and the acylation site in acetylcholinesterase. Chemico-Biological Interactions. 2005;**157-158**:181-189. DOI: 10.1016/j.cbi.2005.10.027

[37] Raba R, Aaviksaar A, Raba M, Siigur J. Cobra venom acetylcholinesterase. Purification and molecular properties. European Journal of Biochemistry. 1979;**96**(1):151-158. DOI: 10.1111/j.1432-1033.1979.tb13024.x

[38] Bourne Y, Renault L, Marchot P. Crystal Structure of Snake Venom acetylcholinesterase in Complex with Inhibitory antibody Fragment Fab410 Bound at the peripheral Site. The Journal of Biological Chemistry. 2015;**290**(3):1522-1535. DOI: 10.1074/jbc.M114.603902

[39] ZELLER EA. The formation of pyrophosphate from adenosine triphosphate in the presence of a snake venom. Arch Biochem. Aug 1950;**28**(1):138-139. PMID: 14771934.

[40] Hassan F, El-Hawary MF, El-Ghazawy A. Acid and alkaline phosphomonoesterases in Egyptian snake venoms. Zeitschrift für Ernährungswissenschaft. 1981;**20**(1):44-54. DOI: 10.1007/BF02027957

[41] Aird SD. Ophidian envenomation strategies and the role of purines. Toxicon. 2002;**40**(4):335-393. DOI: 10.1016/s0041-0101(01)00232-x

[42] Sawynok J. Adenosine and ATP receptors. Handbook of Experimental Pharmacology. 2007;**177**(177):309-328. DOI: 10.1007/978-3-540-33823-9_11

[43] Girish KS, Mohanakumari HP, Nagaraju S, Vishwanath BS, Kemparaju K. Hyaluronidase and protease activities from Indian snake venoms: Neutralization by Mimosa pudica root extract. Fitoterapia. 2004;**75**(3-4):378-380. ISSN 0367-326X. DOI: 10.1016/j.fitote.2004.01.006

[44] Wagstaff SC, Sanz L, Juárez P, Harrison RA, Calvete JJ. Combined snake venomics and venom gland transcriptomic analysis of the ocellated carpet viper, Echis ocellatus. Journal of Proteomics. 2009;**71**(6):609-623. ISSN 1874-3919. DOI: 10.1016/j.jprot.2008.10.003

[45] Wahby AF, El-Sayed ME, Mahdy HA, Salama WH, Abdel-Aty AM, Fahmy AS, et al. Egyptian horned viper Cerastes cerastes venom hyaluronidase: Purification, partial characterization and evidence for its action as a spreading factor. Toxicon. 2012;**60**(8):1380-1389. ISSN 0041-0101. DOI: 10.1016/j.toxicon.2012.08.016

[46] Bordon KC, Perino MG, Giglio JR, Arantes EC. Isolation, enzymatic characterization and antiedematogenic activity of the first reported rattlesnake hyaluronidase from Crotalus durissus terrificus venom. Biochimie. 2012;**94**(12):2740-2748. ISSN 0300-9084. DOI: 10.1016/j.biochi.2012.08.01422940594

[47] Bhavya J, Vineetha MS, Sundaram PM, Veena SM, Dhananjaya BL, More SS. Low-molecular weight hyaluronidase from the venom of *Bungarus caeruleus* (Indian common krait) snake: isolation and partial characterization. Journal of Liquid Chromatography and Related Technologies. 2016;**39**(4):203-208. DOI: 10.1080/10826076.2016.1144203

[48] Harrison RA, Hargreaves A, Wagstaff SC, Faragher B, Lalloo DG. Snake envenoming: A disease of poverty. PLoS Neglected Tropical Diseases. 2009;**3**(12):e569. DOI: 10.1371/journal.pntd.0000569

[49] Eulalio CL, Rodrigues RS, Boldrini-França J, Fonseca FPP, Henrique-Silva F, Homsi-Brandeburgo MI, et al. Molecular cloning of a hyaluronidase from *Bothrops pauloensis*venom gland. Journal of Venomous Animals and Toxins Including Tropical Diseases. 2014;**20**. DOI: 10.1186/1678-9199-20-25

[50] Gopalakrishnakone P, Inagaki H, Vogel Ashis C-W, Mukherjee K, Rahmy TR, editors. Snake Venom. Dordrecht: Springer; 2016

[51] Kini RM. Manjunatha excitement ahead: Structure, function and mechanism of snake venom phospholipase A2 enzymes Toxicon. Toxicon. 2003;**42**(8):827-840. DOI: 10.1016/j.toxicon.2003.11.002

[52] Harris JB, Scott-Davey T. Secreted phospholipases A2 of snake venoms: effects on the peripheral neuromuscular system with comments on the role of phospholipases A2 in disorders of the CNS and their uses in industry. Toxins. 2013;**5**(12):2533-2571. DOI: 10.3390/toxins5122533

[53] Perry BW, Card DC, Mcglothlin JW, Pasquesi GIM, Adams RH, Schield DR, et al. Molecular adaptations for sensing and securing prey and insight into amniote genome diversity from the garter snake genome. Genome Biology and Evolution. 2018;**10**(8):2110-2129. DOI: 10.1093/gbe/evy157

[54] Betzel C, Genov N, Rajashankar KR, Singh TP. Modulation of phospholipase A2 activity generated by molecular evolution. Cellular and Molecular Life Sciences. 1999;**56**(5-6):384-397. DOI: 10.1007/s000180050440

[55] García-Osorio B, Lomonte B, Bénard-Valle M, López de León J, Román-Domínguez L, Mejía-Domínguez NR, et al. Ontogenetic changes in the venom of Metlapilcoatlus nummifer, the Mexican jumping viper. Toxicon. 2020;**184**:204-214. DOI: 10.1016/j.toxicon.2020.06.023

[56] Findrik Z, Geueke B, Hummel W, Vasic-Răcki D. Modelling of L-DOPA enzymatic oxidation catalyzed by L-amino acid oxidases from *Crotalus adamanteus* and *Rhodococcus opacus*. Biochemical Engineering Journal. 2006;**27**(3):275-286. DOI: 10.1016/j.bej.2005.08.022

[57] Fernandes LA, Calderon RG, Mendes MM, Costa TR, Grabner AN, Rodrigues VM, et al. Snake venom

L-amino acid oxidases: Trends in pharmacology and biochemistry. BioMed Research International. 2014;**2014**:196754. 19 pages. DOI: 10.1155/2014/196754

[58] Ande SR, Fussi H, Knauer H, Murkovic M, Ghisla S, Fröhlich KU, et al. Induction of apoptosis in yeast by L-amino acid oxidase from the Malayan pit viper *Calloselasma rhodostoma*. Yeast. 2008;**25**(5):349-357. DOI: 10.1002/yea.1592

[59] Paik WK, Kim S. pH-substrate relationship of l-amino acidoxidases fromsnake venomandrat kidney. Biochimica et Biophysica Acta. 1965;**96**(1):66-74. DOI: 10.1016/0005-2787(65)90610-6

[60] Solis CE, Yarleque EA, et al. Purificaci'on y caracterizaci'on de la L-amino'acido oxidasa del veneno de la serpiente *Bothrops brazili*. Jerg'on shushupe. Revista Peruana de Biología. 1999;**6**:75-84

[61] Stábeli RG, Marcussi S, Carlos GB, Pietro RCLR, Selistre-de-Araújo HS, Giglio JR, et al. Platelet aggregation and antibacterial effects of an l-amino acid oxidase purified from Bothrops alternatus snake venom. Bioorganic & Medicinal Chemistry. 2004;**12**(11):2881-2886. ISSN 0968-0896. DOI: 10.1016/j.bmc.2004.03.049

[62] Kini RM, Koh CY. Metalloproteases affecting blood coagulation, fibrinolysis and platelet aggregation from snake venoms: definition and nomenclature of interaction sites. Toxins. 2016; **8**(10):E284. DOI: 10.3390/toxins8100284

[63] Slagboom J, Kool J, Harrison RA, Casewell NR. Haemotoxic snake venoms: Their functional activity, impact on snakebite victims and pharmaceutical promise. British Journal of Haematology. 2017;**177**(6):947-959. DOI: 10.1111/bjh.14591

[64] Kessler P, Marchot P, Silva M, Servent D. The three-finger toxin fold: A multifunctional structural scaffold able to modulate cholinergic functions. Journal of Neurochemistry. 2017;**142**(Suppl. 2):7-18. DOI: 10.1111/jnc.13975

[65] Reyes-Velasco J, Card DC, Andrew AL, Shaney KJ, Adams RH, Schield DR, et al. Expression of venom gene homologs in diverse python tissues suggests a new model for the evolution of snake venom. Molecular Biology and Evolution. 2015;**32**(1):173-183. DOI: 10.1093/molbev/msu294

[66] Barber CM, Isbister GK, Hodgson WC. Alpha neurotoxins. Toxicon. 2013;**66**:47-58. DOI: 10.1016/j.toxicon.2013.01.019

[67] Sanz L, Pla D, Pérez A, Rodríguez Y, Zavaleta A, Salas M, Lomonte B, Calvete JJ. Venomic analysis of the poorly studied desert coral snake, Micrurus tschudii tschudii, supports the 3FTx/$PLA_2$ dichotomy across Micrurus Venoms. Toxins June 2016;**8**(6):178. DOI: 10.3390/toxins8060178

[68] Vonk FJ, Casewell NR, Henkel CV, Heimberg AM, Jansen HJ, McCleary RJ, et al. The king cobra genome reveals dynamic gene evolution and adaptation in the snake venom system. Proceedings of the National Academy of Sciences of the United States of America. 2013;**110**(51):20651-20656. DOI: 10.1073/pnas.1314702110

[69] Lauridsen LP, Laustsen AH, Lomonte B, Gutiérrez JM. Toxicovenomics and antivenom profiling of the eastern green mamba snake (Dendroaspis angusticeps) (PDF). Journal of Proteomics. 2016;**136**:248-261. DOI: 10.1016/j.jprot.2016.02.003

[70] Changeux JP. The TiPS lecture. The nicotinic acetylcholine receptor: an allosteric protein prototype of

ligand-gated ion channels. Trends in Pharmacological Sciences. 1990;**11**(12):485-492. DOI: 10.1016/0165-6147(90)90049-E

[71] Grant GA, Chiappinelli VA. Kappa-bungarotoxin: Complete amino acid sequence of a neuronal nicotinic receptor probe. Biochemistry. 1985;**24**(6):1532-1537. DOI: 10.1021/bi00327a036

[72] Marchot P, Bourne Y, Prowse CN, Bougis PE, Taylor P. Inhibition of mouse acetylcholinesterase by fasciculin: crystal structure of the complex and mutagenesis of fasciculin. Toxicon. 1998;**36**(11):1613-1622. DOI: 10.1016/S0041-0101(98)00154-8

[73] McDowell RS, Dennis MS, Louie A, Shuster M, Mulkerrin MG, Lazarus RA. Mambin, a potent glycoprotein IIb-IIIa antagonist and platelet aggregation inhibitor structurally related to the short neurotoxins. Biochemistry. 1992;**31**(20):4766-4772. DOI: 10.1021/bi00135a004

[74] Diochot S, Baron A, Salinas M, Douguet D, Scarzello S, Dabert-Gay AS, et al. Black mamba venom peptides target acid-sensing ion channels to abolish pain. Nature. 2012;**490**(7421):552-555. DOI: 10.1038/nature11494

[75] Yang SH, Chien CM, Lu MC, Lu YJ, Wu ZZ, Lin SR. Cardiotoxin III induces apoptosis in K562 cells through a mitochondrial-mediated pathway. Clinical and Experimental Pharmacology & Physiology. 2005;**32**(7):515-520. DOI: 10.1111/j.1440-1681.2005.04223.x

[76] Waqar M, Batool S. *In silico* analysis of binding of neurotoxic venom ligands with acetylcholinesterase for therapeutic use in treatment of Alzheimer's disease. Journal of Theoretical Biology. 2015;**372**:107-117. DOI: 10.1016/j.jtbi.2015.02.028

[77] Blanchet G, Upert G, Mourier G, Gilquin B, Gilles N, Servent D. New α-adrenergic property for synthetic MTbeta and CM-3 three-finger fold toxins from black mamba. Toxicon. 2013;**75**:160-167. DOI: 10.1016/j.toxicon.2013.04.017

[78] Mordvintsev DY, Polyak YL, Levtsova OV, Tourleigh YV, Kasheverov IE, Shaitan KV, et al. A model for short α-neurotoxin bound to nicotinic acetylcholine receptor from *Torpedo californica*: comparison with long-chain α-neurotoxins and α-conotoxins. Computational Biology and Chemistry. 2005;**29**(6):398-411. DOI: 10.1016/j.compbiolchem.2005.08.007

[79] Peng SS, Kumar TK, Jayaraman G, Chang CC, Yu C. Solution structure of toxin b, a long neurotoxin from the venom of the king cobra (*Ophiophagus hannah*). The Journal of Biological Chemistry. 1997;**272**(12):7817-7823. DOI: 10.1074/jbc.272.12.7817

[80] Konshina AG, Krylov NA, Efremov RG. Cardiotoxins: Functional role of local conformational changes. Journal of Chemical Information and Modeling. 2017;**57**(11):2799-2810. DOI: 10.1021/acs.jcim.7b00395

[81] Nguyen TT, Folch B, Létourneau M, Vaudry D, Truong NH, Doucet N, et al. Cardiotoxin-I: an unexpectedly potent insulinotropic agent. Chembiochem. 2012;**13**(12):1805-1812. DOI: 10.1002/cbic.201200081

[82] Rajagopalan N, Pung YF, Zhu YZ, Wong PT, Kumar PP, Kini RM. Beta-cardiotoxin: a new three-finger toxin from *Ophiophagus hannah* (king cobra) venom with β-blocker activity. The FASEB Journal. 2007;**21**(13):3685-3695. DOI: 10.1096/fj.07-8658com

[83] Dufton MJ, Hider RC. Classification of phospholipases A2 according to sequence. Evolutionary and

pharmacological implications. European Journal of Biochemistry. 1983;**137**(3):545-551. DOI: 10.1111/j.1432-1033.1983.tb07860.x

[84] Yang RS, Tang C-H, Chuang W-J, Huang T-H, Peng H-C, Huang T-F, et al. Inhibition of tumor formation by snake venom disintegrin. Toxicon. 2005;**45**(5):661-669. ISSN 0041-0101. DOI: 10.1016/j.toxicon.2005.01.013

[85] Rees B, Samama JP, Thierry JC, Gilibertt M, Fischert J, Schweitzt H, et al. Crystal structure of a snake venom cardiotoxin. Proceedings of the National Academy of Sciences of the United States of America. 1987;**84**:3132-3136

[86] Kumar TKS, Jayaraman G, Lee CS, Arunkumar AI, Sivaraman T, Samuel D, et al. Snake venom cardiotoxins-structure, dynamics, function and folding. Journal of Biomolecular Structure & Dynamics. 1997;**15**(3):431-463. DOI: 10.1080/07391102.1997.10508957

[87] WHO. Snakebite Envenoming. 2021. Available from: https://www.who.int/news-room/fact-sheets/detail/snakebite-envenoming

[88] White J, Warrell D, Eddleston M, Currie BJ, Whyte IM, Isbister GK. Clinical toxinology–where are we now? Journal of Toxicology. Clinical Toxicology. 2003;**41**(3):263-276. DOI: 10.1081/clt-120021112

[89] White J. Elapid snakes. In: Dart RC, editor. Medical Toxicology. Philadelphia: Lippincott Williams & Wilkins; 2004. pp. 1566-1578

[90] Silva A, Isbister GK. Current research into snake antivenoms, their mechanisms of action and applications. Biochemical Society Transactions. 2020;**48**(2):537-546. DOI: 10.1042/BST20190739

[91] Gomes A. Snake venom—an anti arthritis natural product. Al Ameen Journal of Medical Sciences. 2010;**3**:179

[92] Koh CY, Kini RM. From snake venom toxins to therapeutics--cardiovascular examples. Toxicon. 2012;**59**(4):497-506. DOI: 10.1016/j.toxicon.2011.03.017

[93] Vonk FJ, Jackson K, Doley R, Madaras F, Mirtschin PJ, Vidal N. Snake venom: From fieldwork to the clinic: Recent insights into snake biology, together with new technology allowing high-throughput screening of venom, bring new hope for drug discovery. BioEssays. 2011;**33**(4):269-279. DOI: 10.1002/bies.201000117

[94] Waheed H, Moin SF, Choudhary MI. Snake venom: From deadly toxins to Life-Saving Therapeutics. Current Medicinal Chemistry. 2017;**24**(17):1874-1891. DOI: 10.2174/0929867324666170605091546

[95] Smith CG, Vane JR. The discovery of captopril. The FASEB Journal. 2003;**17**(8):788-789. DOI: 10.1096/fj.03-0093life

[96] Peng H, Carretero OA, Vuljaj N, Liao TD, Motivala A, Peterson EL, et al. Angiotensin-converting enzyme inhibitors: A new mechanism of action. Circulation. 2005;**112**(16):2436-2445. DOI: 10.1161/CIRCULATIONAHA.104.528695

[97] Lazarovici P, Marcinkiewicz C, Lelkes PI. From snake venom's disintegrins and C-type lectins to anti-platelet drugs. Toxins. 2019;**11**(5):303. DOI: 10.3390/toxins11050303

[98] Chen Y, Pitzenberger SM, Garsky VM, Lumma PK, Sanyal G, Baum J. Proton NMR assignments and secondary structure of the snake venom protein echistatin. Biochemistry. 1991;**30**(50):11625-11636. DOI: 10.1021/bi00114a004

[99] O'Shea JC, Tcheng JE. Eptifibatide: A potent inhibitor of the platelet

receptor integrin glycoprotein IIb/IIIa. Expert Opinion on Pharmacotherapy. 2002;**3**(8):1199-1210. DOI: 10.1517/14656566.3.8.1199

[100] Vu TT, Stafford AR, Leslie BA, Kim PY, Fredenburgh JC, Weitz JI. Batroxobin binds fibrin with higher affinity and promotes clot expansion to a greater extent than thrombin. The Journal of Biological Chemistry. 2013;**288**(23):16862-16871. DOI: 10.1074/jbc.M113.464750

[101] Lodha A, Kamaluddeen M, Akierman A, Amin H. Role of hemocoagulase in pulmonary hemorrhage in preterm infants: A systematic review. Indian Journal of Pediatrics. 2011;**78**(7):838-844. DOI: 10.1007/s12098-010-0326-4

[102] Ho SJ, Brighton TA. Ximelagatran: Direct thrombin inhibitor. Vascular Health and Risk Management. 2006;**2**(1):49-58. DOI: 10.2147/vhrm.2006.2.1.49

[103] Fukuda K, Doggett T, Laurenzi IJ, Liddington RC, Diacovo TG. The snake venom protein botrocetin acts as a biological brace to promote dysfunctional platelet aggregation. Nature Structural & Molecular Biology. 2005;**12**(2):152-159. DOI: 10.1038/nsmb892

[104] Nakayama D, Ben Ammar Y, Miyata T, Takeda S. Structural basis of coagulation factor V recognition for cleavage by RVV-V. FEBS Letters. 2011;**585**(19):3020-3025. DOI: 10.1016/j.febslet.2011.08.022

[105] Lövgren A. Recombinant snake venom prothrombin activators. Bioengineered. 2013;**4**(3):153-157. DOI: 10.4161/bioe.22676

[106] Lipps BV. Synthetic peptide and uses for same. United States Patent. 2006;**7**(129):334

[107] Minea RO, Helchowski CM, Zidovetzki SJ, Costa FK, Swenson SD, Markland FS Jr. Vicrostatin-an anti-invasive multi-integrin targeting chimeric disintegrin with tumor anti-angiogenic and pro-apoptotic activities. PLoS One. 2010;**5**(6):e10929. DOI: 10.1371/journal.pone.0010929

[108] Hong SY, Lee H, You WK, Chung KH, Kim DS, Song K. The snake venom disintegrin salmosin induces apoptosis by disassembly of focal adhesions in bovine cap- illary endothelial cells. Biochemical and Biophysical Research Communications. 2003;**302**(3):502-508. DOI: 10.1016/s0006-291x(03)00213-4

[109] Pu XC, Wong PTH, Gopalakrishnakone P. A novel analgesic toxin (hannalgesin) from the venom of king cobra (*Ophiophagus hannah*). Toxicon. 1995;**33**(11):1425-1431. DOI: 10.1016/0041-0101(95)00096-5

[110] Perchuc AM, Wilmer M. Diagnostic use of snake venom components in the coagulation laboratory. In: Kini MR, Clemetson KJ, Markland FS, McLane MA, Morita T, editors. Toxins and Hemostasis. Springer: Netherlands; 2010. pp. 747-766

[111] Takacs Z, Nathan S. Animal venoms in medicine. In: *En-* cyclopedia of Toxicology. 3rd ed. Amster- dam. Netherlands: Elsevier; 2014. pp. 252-259

[112] Dutertre S, Lewis RJ. Use of venom peptides to probe ion channel structure and function. The Journal of Biological Chemistry. 2010;**285**(18):13315-13320. DOI: 10.1074/jbc.R109.076596

[113] Dellisanti CD, Yao Y, Stroud JC, Wang ZZ, Chen L. Crystal structure of the extracellular domain of nAChR α1 bound to α-bungarotoxin at 1.94 Å resolution. Nature Neuroscience. 2007;**10**(8):953-962. DOI: 10.1038/nn1942

[114] Bradley KN, Rowan EG, Harvey AL. Effects of mus- carinic toxins MT2 and MT7, from green mamba venom, on m1, M3 and m5 muscarinic receptors expressed in Chi- nese Hamster Ovary cells. Toxicon. 2003;**41**(2):207-215. DOI: 10.1016/s0041-0101(02)00278-7

[115] Mulugeta E, Karlsson E, Islam A, Kalaria R, Mangat H, Winblad B, et al. Loss of muscarinic M 4 recep- tors in hippocampus of Alzheimer patients. Brain Research. 2003;**960**(1):259-262

Chapter 2

# Snake Venom and Therapeutic Potential

*Mamdouh Ibrahim Nassar*

## Abstract

Many active secretions produced by animals have been employed in the development of new drugs to treat diseases such as hypertension and cancer. Snake venom toxins contributed significantly to the treatment of many medical conditions. Snake venoms are the secretion of venomous snakes, which are synthesized and stored in specific venom glands. Many toxins from snake venom are investigated and formulated into drugs for the treatment of conditions such as cancer, hypertension, and thrombosis. Most of the venoms are complex mixture of a number of proteins, peptides, enzymes, toxins and non-protein inclusions. Cytotoxic effects of snake venom have potential to degrade and destroy tumor cells. Different species have different types of venom, which depends upon its species, geographical location, its habitat, climate and age. The purpose of this chapter is to review focusing on the therapeutic potential of snake venoms and to establish a scientific basis for diseases treatment particular antitumor.

**Keywords:** snake venom, cancer therapy, diseases treatment

## 1. Introduction

Snake venoms are the secretion of venomous snakes, which are synthesized and stored in special glands. The venom were synthesized and stored into the base of channeled or tubular fangs through which it is ejected. Most of the venoms are complex mixture of a number of proteins, peptides, enzymes, toxins and non-protein inclusions [1]. Some of snake venom possess biological effects on various functions, such as blood coagulation and pressure, regulation, and transmission of nerve impulses. These venoms have been studied and developed by researchers for use as pharmacological or diagnostic tools, and even drugs. Snake venom is a therapeutic agent for various diseases due to its physiologically active components [2]. More specifically, cobra venom has been used historically in Ayurveda in the treatment of arthritis and other chronic diseases [3].

Chinese physicians are implementing the use of snake venom products to treat stroke patients, and research has been conducted surrounding its analgesic, anti-cancerous and anti-inflammatory effects [2]. Cytotoxic effects of snake venom have potential to degrade and destroy tumor cells [4]. There are basically three types of snake venom according to its effects [5, 6]. (a) Hemotoxic venoms, which affects cardiovascular system and blood functions, (b) cytotoxic venoms targets specific cellular sites or muscles and (c) neurotoxic venoms harms nervous system of human body. The families, Elapidae and Viperidae, are large majority of the research done surrounding the medical application of snake venom involves species within these groups. Both elapids and vipers are front fanged snakes that belong to the superfamily Colubroidea. Notable species of the elapid family are cobras of the genus *Naja,* and a well-researched species in the viper family is *Crotalus durissus terrificus.*

Snake venom components caused retardation of growth of cancerous cells due to its therapeutic activity, potency for many diseases and disorders [7]. Many excellent publications characterized use of venoms for the treatment of various therapeutic conditions such as human diseases, cancer and inflammation [8, 9].

## 2. Components of snake venom

Snake venoms are complex mixtures; mainly it has proteins, which have enzymatic activities, inorganic cations, calcium, potassium, magnesium, zinc, nickel, cobalt, iron, and manganese. Zinc is necessary for anti-cholinesterase activity; calcium is required for activation of enzyme like phospholipase. Some snake venoms also contain carbohydrate, lipid, biogenic amines, and free amino acids [10].

## 3. Snake enzymes

Proteins found in snake venom include toxins, neurotoxins, nontoxic proteins, and many enzymes, especially hydrolytic ones. Enzymes are protein in nature including digestive hydrolases, L-amino-acid oxidase, phospholipases, thrombin-like pro-coagulant, and kallikrein-like serine proteases and metalloproteinases (hemorrhagins), which damage vascular endothelium.

Phosphodiesterases enzyme interfere with the prey's cardiac system, mainly to lower the blood pressure. Phospholipase A2 causes hemolysis by lysing the phospholipid cell membranes of red blood cells [2]. Amino acid oxidases and proteases are used for digestion. Also amino acid oxidase triggers some other enzymes and is responsible for the yellow color of the venom. Hyaluronidase enzymes increases tissue permeability to accelerate the absorption of other enzymes into tissues **Table 1**.

## 4. Polypeptide toxins

Pllypeptides include cytotoxins, cardiotoxins, and postsynaptic neurotoxins (such as α-bungarotoxin and α-Cobratoxin), which bind to acetylcholine receptors at neuromuscular junctions. Also polypeptides contains metals, peptides, lipids, nucleosides, carbohydrates, amines, and oligopeptides. Chemical composition variations of snake venom due to geographical and Ontogenic of the different species [3].

### 4.1 Proteolytic enzymes

These enzymes catalyze the breakdown of tissue proteins and peptides. They are also known as peptide hydrolases, protease, endopeptidases and proteinases. Some metal ions of the proteolytic enzymes help in catalysis involved in the activity of certain venom proteases and phospholipases [10].

### 4.2 Arginine ester hydrolase

Non-cholinesterase enzymes, it causes hydrolysis of the ester or peptide linkage, to which an arginine residue contributes the carboxyl group. This activity was found

| Type | Name | Origin species |
|---|---|---|
| Oxidoreductases | Dehydrogenase Lactate | Elapidae |
| | L-amino-acid oxidase | All species |
| | Catalase | All species |
| Transferases | Alanine amino transferase | |
| Hydrolases | Phospholipase A2 | All species |
| | Lysophospholipase | Elapidae, Viperidae |
| | Acetylcholinesterase | Elapidae |
| | Alkaline phosphatase | *Bothrops atrox* |
| | Acid phosphatase | *Deinagkistrodon acutus* |
| | 5′-nucleotidase | All species |
| | Phosphodiesterase | All species |
| | Deoxyribonuclease | All species |
| | Ribonuclease 1 | All species |
| | Adenosine triphosphatase | All species |
| | Amylase | All species |
| | Hyaluronidase | All species |
| | NAD-nucleotidase | All species |
| | Kininogenase | Viperidae |
| | Factor X activator | Viperidae, Crotalinae |
| | Heparinase | Crotalinae |
| | α-Fibrinogenase | Viperidae, Crotalinae |
| | β-Fibrinogenase | Viperidae, Crotalinae |
| | α-β-Fibrinogenase | *Bitis gabonica* |
| | Fibrinolytic enzyme | Crotalinae |
| | Prothrombin activator | Crotalinae |
| | Collagenase | Viperidae |
| | Elastase | Viperidae |
| Lyases | Glucosaminate ammonia-lyase | |

**Table 1.**
*Main enzymes of snake venom [1].*

in snake, crotalid, viperid and some sea snake venoms [10]. Several arginine ester hydrolases have been isolated from the venoms of different snake species. These enzymes eventually showed fibrinogenolytic, caseinolytic, bradykinin releasing or edema-inducing activities. Most of them are serine proteases [11].

### 4.3 Thrombin-like enzymes

Snake venom thrombin-like enzymes (SVTLEs) constitute the major portion (10–24%) of snake venom and these are the second most abundant enzymes present in the crude venom. These enzymes are glycoprotein in nature, and act as defibrinating anticoagulants in vivo, whereas in vitro they clot plasma, heparinised plasma and purified fibrinogen. It used as therapeutic agent for the treatment of various diseases such as congestive heart failure, ischemic stroke, thrombotic disorders.

Thrombin like enzymes such as crotalase, agkistrodon, ancrod and batroxobin can be purified from different snake venoms [12].

### 4.4 Collagenase

Collagenase enzymes are proteinase in nature that digests collagen and mesenteric collagen fibers [13]. Collagenase are also compounds of snake venoms, may induce disruption of retinal veins that, in turn, result in retinal hemorrhage. Collagenase could as drug leading to the development of new treatments due to its proteolytic properties in their pathophysiology.

### 4.5 Hyaluronidase

hyaluronidase beyond its role as a spreading factor venom it deserves to be explored as a therapeutic target for inhibiting the systemic distribution of venom bite. It acts upon connective tissues and decreases their viscosity, catalyzes the cleavage of internal glycoside bonds. Hyaluronidase enzyme has been found to be ubiquitously distributed in snake venoms. Hyaluronidase enzyme by itself is non-toxic and has long been known as 'spreading factor'. The breakdown in the hyaluronic barrier allows some other fractions of venom to penetrate the organ tissues [2].

### 4.6 Phospholipase

Phospholipases are enzymes that hydrolyse glycerophospholipids. It catalyzes the calcium dependent hydrolysis of the 2-acyl ester bond thereby producing free fatty acids and lysophospho lipid. Neurotoxic phospholipases $A_2$ ($PLA_2$s) very large superfamily of enzymes composed of 16 groups within six major types. $PLA_2$s can bind to and hydrolyse membrane phospholipids of the motor nerve terminal to cause degeneration of the nerve terminal and skeletal muscle. PLA2 can also cause hydrolysis of membrane phospholipids, and liberation of some bioactive products [14]. The biotechnological effectively of PLA2 inhibitors may support the therapeutic potential with antiophidian activity.

### 4.7 Phosphodiestsrase

Snake poisonous venom phosphodiesterase is a zinc metalloenzyme that share a number of mechanistic features with the nucleotidyl transferases. Zinc of this enzyme is activated by magnesium, and catalyze $\alpha$-$\beta$ phosphoryl bond cleavage. Phosphodiesterase releases 5-mononucleotide chain act as an exonucleotidase, thereby affecting DNA and RNA functions [15].

### 4.8 Acetylcholinesterase

Snake acetylcholinesterase in general is found in cobra and sea snake but absent in viperid and crotalid venoms. It plays a role in cholinergic transmission which located at the neuro-muscular junction of vertebrates.

## 5. Pharmaceutical assessment of snake venom

Some of snake venom components which have spurred the development of novel pharmaceutical compounds. Snake venom are investigated for the treatment of many diseases as cancer, hypertension, and thrombosis. Venoms of rattlesnakes and other crotalids produce alterations in resistance of blood vessels, changes in blood cells and coagulation and changes in cardiac and pulmonary dynamics. Also it may cause alterations in nervous system and respiratory system [16–20]. The potency of venom and its effect on human depend on the type and amount of venom injected and the site where it is deposited. Different other parameters and therapeutic derived such as hypotension and nerve shock and fall in blood pressure and varying degree of shock followed by a decrease in heamatocrit values are associated with snake venom [21–23].

## 6. Snake venom in medicine

Snake venoms are a cocktail of potent compounds which specifically and avidly target numerous essential molecules with high efficacy. The individual effects of all venom toxins integrate into lethal dysfunctions of almost any organ system. Such toxin mimetic may help in influencing a specific body function pharmaceutically for the sake of man's health. Such snake toxin-derived mimetic are in clinical use, trials, or consideration for further pharmaceutical exploitation, especially in the fields of hemostasis, thrombosis, coagulation, and metastasis. Snake venom has great potential use as a medicine, because of all the compounds it contains, and their specific actions. Two analgesics derive from cobra venom; Cobroxin is used like morphine to block nerve transmission, and Nyloxin reduces severe arthritis pain [24]. Arvin compound from *Malayan pitviper* is an effective anticoagulant. Venom components allow researchers to develop novel drugs for treatment many diseases such as, nerve epilepsy, multiple sclerosis, myasthenia gravis, Parkinson's disease, and poliomyelitis, musculoskeletal disease [24].

## 7. Snake venom and diseases treatment

Given that snake venom contains many biologically active ingredients, some may be useful to treat disease [25].

Phospholipases type A2 (PLA2s) from the Tunisian vipers *Cerastes cerastes* and *Macrovipera lebetina* have been found to have antitumor activity [26, 27]. PLA2s hydrolyze phospholipids, thus could act on bacterial cell surfaces, providing novel antimicrobial activities [28]. The analgesic activity of many snake venom proteins has been long known [29, 30] and the main challenge is how to deliver protein to the nerve cells.

## 8. Serotherapy of snake venom

Serotherapy using antivenom is a common current treatment, both adaptive immunity and serotherapy are specific to the type of snake; venom with identical physiological action do not cross-neutralize [31, 32].

## 9. Snake venom therapy of hepatocellular carcinoma

Hepatocellular carcinoma (HCC) represents up to 90% of all liver malignancies. Recently, the World Health Organization (WHO) reported that HCC is the fifth most common tumor worldwide, and the second most common cause of cancer-associated deaths. For the majority of advanced HCC cases, curative treatments are not possible, and the prognosis is dismal because of underlying cirrhosis as well as poor tumor response to standard chemotherapy. For patients with advanced HCC, the only approved molecular targeted therapy is sorafenib (SOR), the first orally active multi-kinase inhibitor. It provides only temporary therapeutic efficacy by increasing the survival rate by approximately 3 months [33]. Besides, a great inter-individual variation in the pharmacokinetics of SOR, due to systemic overexposure, has contributed to its toxicity [34, 35]. Therapeutic approaches to identify and develop novel compounds such as snake venom components are urgent to have potential ability for cancer treatment [36]. Moreover, better finding alternative natural safe, and better ways to treat cancer with less toxicity and deteriorated effect on normal cells is highly desirable [37].

The combining snake venoms (SVs) could synergistically enhance the antiproliferative effects at low doses on liver cancer cells (HepG2). In such Research the gene expression for apoptotic, inflammatory, antioxidant and cell cycle regulator was determined [38].

Varies compounds from venomous animals such as spiders, scorpions, snakes, caterpillars, centipedes, wasp, bees, toads, ants, and frogs have largely shown biotechnological and pharmacological applications against many diseases including cancer [39–42]. Venoms obtained from snakes were reported to exhibit a cytotoxic effect against tumor cells [26]. This potency is due to inhibiting cell proliferation, promoting cell death through activating the apoptotic mechanisms [43, 44]. Meanwhile snake venom increased cytochrome-c production, modulating the expression levels of proteins that controlling the cell cycle, and treat triggering damages in the cell membranes [45–47].

The complex mixtures of snake venom, L-amino acid oxidase (LAAO) are a effect as anticancer therapeutic activity and through the induction of oxidative stress in cancer cells [48]. L-amino acid oxidase (LAAO) has been reported to exhibit a potent anti-tumor activity to different cancer cell lines including [49]. LAAO can selectively bind to the cancer cell surface at specific phospholipid compositions to deliver the hydrogen peroxide [47–50]. LAAO mediates its cytotoxicity to the cell surface and produces $H_2O_2$ [49, 51, 52]. Moreover studies are confirmed this safer effect on animal models [38]. In terms of cytotoxicity, combined administration of LAAO with SOR has reduced the cell death on normal liver cells THLE-2 as compared to a single administration [38]. On the other hand the administration of LAAO and SV alone or in combination with SOR has significantly induced cell death and apoptosis in HepG2 cells as compared to control untreated cells [53]. Additionally, [54] showed that the LAAO isolated from *Ophiophagus hannah* venom selectively kills cancer cells via the apoptotic pathway by regulating the caspase 3, 7 activity but is non-toxic to normal cells. One of the consequences of the excessive damage caused by the reactive oxygen species (ROS) is changes in mitochondrial membrane permeability causing $Ca^{+2}$ overload that result in cytochrome c release and apoptotic death [55].

## 10. Therapeutic effects of snake venom on rheumatoid

Rheumatoid arthritis (RA) is a chronic, systemic autoimmune disease in which the immune system primarily attacks healthy tissue of synovial joints (NIH). The disease affects between 0.5–1.0% of the developed world population, and is a significant cause of disability [56]. The primary characteristic of RA is the progressive destruction and inflammation of synovial joints, most commonly in metacarpophalangeal, proximal interphalangeal, metatarsophalangeal, wrist, and knee joints. Articular manifestations include symmetric joint swelling, tenderness, stiffness, and motion impairment, and general symptoms such as fevers, fatigue, weight loss, and discomfort are also common [57].

Snake venom has been used for treatment of rheumatoid arthritis and pain management. Venom from the families *Elapidae* and *Viperidae* have been shown to have anti-inflammatory and analgesic effects. Snake venom has anti-inflammatory effects by reducing levels of pro- inflammatory cytokines and increasing levels of anti-inflammatory cytokines [58]. Additionally, snake venom can reduce structural damage from prolonged inflammation by acting as a (tumor necrosis factor alpha), TNF-alpha blocker, and by inhibiting the proliferation of fibroblast-like synoviocytes. The mechanisms of snake venom pain modulation seen in murine pain models follow the cholinergic and opioidergic systems. Analgesic findings involving the cholinergic system concluded not only that the effects of snake venom have similar effects to morphine, but also that no withdrawal symptoms were observed after administration of venom stopped. These results show incredible promise for a non-addictive analgesic that could be used for pain management in rheumatoid arthritis patients [58].

A study found that while the general health status of RA patients in Norway improved between the years of 1994 and 2001, alleviation of pain remained the highest priority in both cohorts [59]. In another study, 88% of participants selected pain as their top priority for improvement during a year of treatment [60]. Pain scores are also disproportionately greater in women, minorities, and those with lesser levels of education, and pain is a top contributor to emotional health in RA patients [61, 62].

One of the main treatments for pain in RA patients is the administration of disease modifying antirheumatic drugs (DMARDs), which act peripherally to reduce the inflammatory response and the pain associated with it. Additionally, non-steroidal anti-inflammatory drugs (NSAIDs) such as ibuprofen and naproxen are often suggested to patients to manage their pain. These medications can be coupled with over the counter medications such as acetaminophen to further alleviate pain. When the combination of NSAID and acetaminophen administration has failed to provide relief, weak opioids are considered [63]. Therapies for RA have generally shifted focus from symptom management to the treatment of underlying inflammation that causes the symptoms [64]. Biologic disease modifying drugs are act to reduce immune responses in the body such as TNF inhibitors are used to block tumor necrosis factor (a proinflammatory cytokine) activity. Similarly, Abatacept prevents the overactivity of T cells, and Tocilluzumab inhibits the activity of another proinflammatory protein, IL-6 [65, 66].

Mechanical and thermal hyperalgesia have been found to be suppressed in several murine models with the administration of snake venom. Inflammation can also affect central pain processing, so a decrease in inflammation with snake venom could positively affect central pain and sensitization as well. The effects of snake venom from elapids and vipers on cholinergic and opioidergic mechanisms of pain are arguably the most promising relevant to treating rheumatoid arthritis. In one study, snake venom acting on cholinergic receptors to produce analgesia was found to be just as effective as morphine, with a longer lasting effect [67]. A handful of studies have utilized venom from elapids, particularly the species *Naja kaouthia* and *Naja naja,* in murine arthritis models to study the anti-inflammatory and anti-arthritic properties of the venom or its specific components [68]. Observed the effects of NN-32, a cytotoxic protein from *N. naja* venom, on arthritic rats. It was found that while arthritic rats showed significantly increased levels of inflammatory cytokines TNF-α, IL-17, and cytokine-induced neutrophil chemoattractant 1 (CINC-1, a rat cytokine (homolog of IL-8) with hyperalgesic properties) compared to non-arthritic control rats, NN-32 treatment significantly decreased levels of these cytokines. Another study by the same researchers found that IL-10 levels were decreased in adjuvant induced arthritic rats, but the levels were significantly restored when treated by *N. kaouthia* venom [69].

Produced similar results using cobratoxin, a neurotoxin from a *Naja* cobra, on complete Freund's adjuvant (CFA) induced arthritis rats [70]. The arthritic rats showed increased serum levels of (tumor necrosis factor) TNF-α, IL-1, and IL-2, and decreased levels of IL-10. With the cobratoxin treatment, the rats exhibited lower proinflammatory cytokine levels, and a reversal of the CFA induced IL-10 decrease [69]. Found similar results with neurotoxin-NNA, another peptide from *N. naja atra*: Treatment with the peptide exhibited a dose dependent decrease in TNF-α and IL-1β levels in rat models of inflammation. These studies add to the evidence that cobra venom could modulate the production of inflammatory cytokines in RA and subsequently reduce inflammatory pain.

Compared the effects of cobratoxin from *N. naja atra* to dexamethasone, a corticosteroid that relieves inflammation. This revealed the dexamethasone administered to arthritic rats showed greater effects on acute inflammation than the cobrotoxin, but inhibition of the long-term inflammatory process (observed by a decrease of cytokines IL-6, TNF-α, and IL- 1β) was strong in both. The maintenance of the levels suggests that orally administered CTX has anti-inflammatory properties by decreasing pro-inflammatory cytokine levels and maintaining pro-inflammatory cytokine levels. Rats treated with CTX showed slightly greater anti-inflammatory and analgesic effects, suggesting the potential for components of venom to function as NSAIDs [69].

## 11. Snake venom therapy of joint destruction

The use of tumor necrosis factor (TNF) blockers, a more recent therapeutic option for RA, provides a correlation between the cytokine TNF-α and bone erosion. Several studies have found that the five TNF blockers that are currently in use have all been correlated with continued inhibition of bone erosion [71]. The positive effect of TNF inhibitors provides evidence that a decrease in the cytokine TNF-α could have beneficial effects on reducing not only initial inflammatory pain but also pain induced by bone erosion and other structural changes. Additionally, the anti arthritic and anti inflammatory activity of NN-32, a cytotoxic protein from Indian spectacle cobra snake *(Naja naja)* venom showed significant decrease in physical and urinary parameters, serum enzymes, serum cytokines levels as compared to arthritic control group of rats. NN-32 treatment recovered carrageenan induced inflammation [72]; Cobratoxin (CTX), the long-chain α-neurotoxin from *Thailand cobra* venom, has been demonstrated to have analgesic action in rodent pain models [73]. Structural changes of bone and cartilage are a hallmark of inflammatory joint diseases such as rheumatoid arthritis (RA), psoriatic arthritis (PsA), and ankylosing spondylitis (AS) [74, 75] found that cobrotoxin from *N. naja atra* venom inhibited the activation of nuclear factor kappa B (NF-κB). NF-κB is a transcriptional factor that plays a role in inflammation by expressing pro-inflammatory cytokines, including TNF-α, and inhibition of NF-κB has been shown to delay progression of joint destruction in animal arthritis models. Another study also found that cobrotoxin has an inhibitory effect on NF-κB activation, which led to decreased levels of TNF-α [76]. These studies indicate that cobra venom can decrease proinflammatory cytokine levels, affecting as anti-inflammatory properties pain associated with physical destruction of the joint. These properties could reduce both peripheral and central inflammation, and potentially prevent further joint damage and sensitization of nerves [77].

## 12. Therapeutic potential of snake venom on cancer

The anti-cancer potential of snake venom depend on its protein peptides and enzymes which bind to cancer cell membranes, affecting the migration and proliferation of these cells [78].

Cancer is characterized by uncontrolled cell division, cell transformation, and escape of apoptosis, invasion, angiogenesis and metastasis. Induction of apoptosis is the most important mechanism of many anticancer agents. Snake integrins are important in cell adhesion, cell migration, tissue organization, cell growth, hemostasis and inflammatory responses, so they are in the study for the development of drugs for the treatment of cancer [53]. The induction of the apoptosis manifests the control on the tumor size and number of tumor cells hence establishing the application of apoptosis inducers as vital components in the treatment of cancer [55].

Isolation and purification of L-amino acid oxidases (LAAOs) from *Bothrops leucurus* (Bl-LAAO) and cobra was effected on platelet function and cytotoxicity [79, 80]. The mechanism of this enzyme action may be related to the inhibition of thymidine incorporation and an interaction with DNA [81]. Also different tumor cell lines were found to susceptible from lytic action and from synthetic peptide. Also NN-32 showed cytotoxicity on EAC cells, increased survival time of inoculated EAC mice, reduced solid tumor volume and weight. NN-32 increased proapoptotic protein [82]. Pharmacokinetics effect of cytotoxin from Chinese cobra (*N. naja atra*) venom was studied on rabbits [49]. Plasma levels of the cytotoxin were analyzed by a biotinavidin enzyme-linked immunosorbent assay.

The extraction of specific protein Okinawa Habu apoxin protein-1 (OHAP-1) from Okinawa Habu venom studied for its toxic effects [83]. In this study, OHAP-1 could induce apoptosis in some glioma cell. Also the apoptotic effect of OHAP-1 on malignant glioma cells could be through the generation of intracellular ROS and p53 protein expression. Antitumor activity using snake venom (*Lapemis curtus*) caused decreasing of Hep2 tumor volume and considered as an important indicator of reduction of tumor burden [84]. Cardiotoxin III (CTX III), was isolated from *N. naja atra* venom, and reported its anticancer activity [85]. The anti-tumor potential as well as its cytotoxicity and hemolysis activity was occurred as a galactoside-binding lectin which isolated from *B. leucurus* venom [86]. Purification of BjcuL, a lectin from *Bothrops jararacussu* venom was observed its cytotoxic effects to gastric carcinoma cells. This confirmed cytotoxicity of BJcuL on tumor cells mainly by altering cell adhesion and through induction of apoptosis [87].

## 13. Anti-microbial potency of snake venom

Snakes venoms were assayed in order to investigate their antimicrobial activities giving promising results [88]. Since 1930s, cobra venom has been used to treat various diseases like asthma, polio, multiple sclerosis, rheumatism, severe pain and trigeminal neuralgia. Among antimicrobial components that have been isolated from snake venom are (i) L-amino acid oxidase (LAAO), and (ii) phospholipase A2 (PLA2) [89]. The LAAO antibacterial action appears to result from hydrogen peroxide generated by the oxidative action of the enzymes, as the effect is abolished in the presence of hydrogen peroxide scavengers such as catalase [10, 90–93]. Also antimicrobial peptides including cathelicidins, nerve growth factor and omwaprin have been isolated from various venomous snake species [94–96]. The antibacterial effects of cobra venom LAAO were affected against strains including *S. aureus, S. epidermidis, P. aeruginosa, Klebsiella pneumoniae*, *E. coli*, gram-positive and negative bacteria [92, 97]. Purified L-amino acid oxidase from *Bothrops pauloensis* snake venom had bactericidal activities [98, 99].

Electron microscopic assessments of both Gram-positive and Gram-negative bacterial strains suggested that the $H_2O_2$ produced by LAO induced bacterial membrane rupture and consequently loss of cytoplasmatic content [100, 101]. Akbu-LAAO an L-amino acid oxidase isolated from the venom of *Agkistrodon blomhoffii ussurensis* snake exhibited a strong bacteriostasis effect on *S. aureus* [102].

The most mode of action involved in the bactericidal activity of LAAOs is that $H_2O_2$ causes oxidative stress in the target cell, triggering disorganization of the plasma membrane and cytoplasm and consequent cell death **Table 2** [103, 104].

### 13.1 Anti-microbial activity of phospholipase A2 (PLA2)

Phospholipase has antimicrobial activity against *E. coli* and *S. aureus* as well as the Gram-positive bactericidal activity of sPLA(2)-I [105]. Also Phospholipases A2 (PLA2S) isolated from *C. durissus terrificus* venom showed antimicrobial activity against *Xanthomonas axonopodis* pv. Passiflorae **Table 3** [106].

| Snake species | Antibacterial component | Effective against |
|---|---|---|
| *Bothrops mattogrosensis* | BmLAAO | Gram positive and negative bacteria |
| *Ophiophagus Hannah* | King cobra L-amino acid oxidase (Oh-LAAO) | Gram positive and negative bacteria |
| *B. alternatus* | Balt-LAAO-I | *E. coli* and *S. aureus* |
| *Daboia russellii siamensis* | DRS-LAAO | *S. aureus* (ATCC 25923), *P. aeruginosa* (ATCC 27853) and *E. coli* (ATCC 25922). |
| King cobra venom | LAAO | *S. aureus, S. epidermidis, P. aeruginosa, K. pneumoniae*, and *E. coli* |
| *B. pauloensis* | Bp-LAAO | Not specific |
| *Bothriechis schlegelii* | BsLAAO | *S. aureus* and *Acinetobacter baumannii* |
| *Naja naja oxiana* | LAAO | *B. subtilis* and *E. coli* |
| *Crotalus durissus cascavella* | Casca LAAO | (*Xanthomonas axonopodis pv passiflorae*) and *S. mutans* |
| *Crotalus durissus cumanensis* | CdcLAAO | *S. aureus* and *A. baumannii* |
| *Vipera lebetina* | LAAO | Gram-negative and Gram-positive bacteria |
| *Agkistrodon blomhoffiiussurensis* | Akbu-LAAO | *S. aureus* |
| *Trimeresurus mucrosquamatus* | TM-LAO | *E. coli, S. aurues* and *B. dysenteriae* |
| *Trimeresurus jerdonii* | TJ-LAO | *E. coli, S. aureus, P. aeruginosa*, and *Bacillus megaterium*. |
| *Bothrops marajoensis* | BmarLAAO | *S. aureus*, and *P. aeruginosa* |
| *Bothrops jararaca* | LAAO | *S. aureus* |
| *Agkistrodon haly Pallas* | LAAO | *E coli* K12D31 |
| B. leucurus | BleuLAAO | S. aureus |

**Table 2.**
*Anti-bacterial profile of various snake venom LAAOs [88].*

| Snake species | Antibacterial component | Effective against |
|---|---|---|
| *Bungarus fasciatus* | BFPA | *E. coli* and *S. aureus* |
| Agkistrodon spp | AgkTx-II | *S. aureus*, *P. vulgaris* and *Burkholderia pseudomallei* |
| *Echis carinatus* | EcTx-I | *Enterobacter aerogenes*, *E. coli*, *P. vulgaris*, *P. mirabilis*, *P. aeruginosa* and *S. aureus* |
| *Vipera berus berus* | VBBPLA2 | *B. subtilis* |
| *Bothrops asper* | PLA2 myotoxins | *S. typhimurium* and *S. aureus* |
| *Porthidium nasutum* | PnPLA2 | *S. aureus* |

**Table 3.**
*Antibacterial profile of various snake venom Phospholipae A2s [88].*

### 13.2 Antimicrobial activity of peptides

Peptides are have a critical defense against all kinds of microorganisms, bacteria, fungi, and viruses. Peptides play an important role in the bactericidal effect. Antimicrobial peptides can be divided into four structural groups known as α-helical, β-sheet, α-hairpin, and extended peptides [107].

### 13.3 Cathelicidin

Cathelicidin-BF found in the venom of the snake *Bungarus fasciatus* in treating *Salmonella typhimurium* infection. Cathelicidins are a family of antimicrobial peptides acting as multifunctional effectors molecule in innate immunity. Cathelicidin-BF had been purified from the snake venoms of *B. fasciatus* (BF) and it was the first identified cathelicidin antimicrobial peptide in reptiles [88]. *S. epidermidis*, was also effectively killed by Cathelicidin-BF [108, 109].

Cathelicidin-BF is active against Salmonella infected-mice and it showed strong antibacterial activity against various bacteria [110]. Cathelicidin from the venom of *B. fasciatus* has antibacterial activity against drug-resistant *E. coli, P. aeruginosa*, and *S. aureus*. Also cathelicidin BF-30 had stronger antimicrobial activities against a broad spectrum of microorganisms [111].

## 14. Conclusions

Snake venoms are the complex mixtures of several biologically active proteins, peptides, enzymes, and organic and inorganic compounds.

Snake venoms are very important agents for many types of diseases as well as antimicrobial, anti-inflammation, anti-rheumatoid and cancer therapy. Snake venoms acts by inhibiting cell proliferation and promoting cell death by different means: induction of apoptosis in cancer cell, increasing $Ca^{2+}$ influx; inducing cytochrome C release; decreasing or increasing the expression of proteins that control cell cycle; leading to damage of cell membranes. Snake venoms contain many components that act on the peripheral nervous system for killing or immobilizing prey. All the above mentioned attracted our attention to develop of a new drugs from snake venoms will be useful as therapeutic agents of many diseases.

## Author details

Mamdouh Ibrahim Nassar
Faculty of Science, Cairo University, Egypt

*Address all correspondence to: mmnassar2002@yahoo.com

## References

[1] Leon G, Sanchez L, Hernandez A, Villalta M, Herrera M, Segura A, et al. Immune response towards snake venoms. Inflammation & Allergy Drug Targets. 2011;**10**:381-398

[2] Sudhakar KA, Dumantraj AR, Sonali C. A review on Snake venom: An unrevealed medicine for human ailments: Great scope for pharmaceutical research. International Journal of Research in Ayurveda and Pharmacy. 2017;**8**(2):35-41. DOI: 10.7897/2277-4343.08280

[3] Gomes A, Bhattacharya S, Chakraborty M, Bhattacharjee P, Mishra R, Gomes A. Anti-arthritic activity of Indian monocellate cobra (*Naja kaouthia*) venom on adjuvant induced arthritis. Toxicon. 2010;**55** (2-3):670-673. DOI: 10.1016/j.toxicon.2009.10.007

[4] Marsh N, Williams V. Practical applications of snake venom toxins in haemostasis. Toxicon. 2005;**45**:1171-1181

[5] Jin H, Varner J. Integrins: Roles in cancer development and as treatment targets. British Journal of Cancer. 2004;**90**:561-565

[6] Debatin KM, Krammerr P. Death receptors in chemotherapy and cancer. Oncogene. 2004;**23**:2950-2966

[7] Kalam Y, Isbister GK, Mirtschin P, Hodgson WC, Konstantakopoulos N. Validation of a cell-based assay to differentiate between the cytotoxic effects of elapid snake venoms. Journal of Pharmacological and Toxicological Methods. 2011;**63**:137-142

[8] Gomes A, Bhattacharjee P, Mishra R, Biswas AK, Dasgupta SC, Giri B. Anticancer potential of animal venoms and toxins. Indian Journal of Experimental Biology. 2010;**48**:93-103

[9] Santos MMDV, Santana CD, Giglio JR, Da Silva RJ, Sampaio SV, Soares AM, et al. Antitumoural effect of an *L*-amino acid oxidase isolated from *Bothrops jararaca* snake venom. Basic & Clinical Pharmacology & Toxicology. 2008;**102**:533-542

[10] Kitchens CS, Eskin TA. Fatality in a case of envenomation by *Crotalus adamanteus* initially successfully treated with polyvalent ovine antivenom followed by recurrence of defibrinogenation syndrome. Journal of Medical Toxicology. 2008;**4**:180-183

[11] Pmdrio-Escarso SH, Soares AM, Rodrigues VM, Mancin AC, Reis ML, Ballejo G, et al. Isolation and characterization of an arginine ester hydrolase from *Bothrops jararacussu* venom which induces contractions of the isolated rat uterus. Biochemistry and Molecular Biology International. 1999;**47**(4):699-706

[12] Ullah A, Masood R, Ali I, Ullah K, Ali H, Akbar H, et al. Thrombin-like enzymes from snake venom: Structural characterization and mechanism of action. International Journal of Biological Macromolecules. 2018; **114**(788):811. DOI: 10.1016/j.ijbiomac.2018.03.164

[13] Chu CW, Tsai TS, Tsai IH, Lin YS, Tu MC. Prey envenomation does not improve digestive performance in Taiwanese pit vipers (*Trimeresurus gracilis* and *T. stejnegeri stejnegeri*). Comparative Biochemistry & Physiology. 2009;**152A**:579-585

[14] Wuster W, Peppin L, Pook CE, Walker DE. A nesting of vipers: Phylogeny, historical biogeography and patterns of diversification of the Viperidae (Squamata: Serpentes). Molecular Phylogenetics and Evolution. 2008;**49**:445-459

[15] Tsai CH, Yang SH, Chien CM, Lu MC, Lo CS, Lin YH, et al. Mechanisms of cardiotoxin III-induced apoptosis in human colorectal cancer colo205 cells. Clinical and Experimental Pharmacology & Physiology. 2006; **33**:177-182

[16] Gallacci M, Cavalcante WLG. Understanding the *in vitro* neuromuscular activity of snake venom Lys49 phospholipase A2 homologues. Toxicon. 2010;**55**:1-11

[17] Marcussi S, Sant'Ana CD, Oliveira CZ, Rueda AQ, Menaldo DL, Beleboni RO, et al. Snake venom phospholipase A2 inhibitors: Medicinal chemistry and therapeutic potential. Current Topics in Medicinal Chemistry. 2007;**7**:743-756

[18] Gutierrez JM, Alexandra R, Escalante T, Díaz C. Hemorrhage induced by snake venom metalloproteinases: Biochemical and biophysical mechanisms involved in microvessel damage. Toxicon. 2005;**45**:997-1011

[19] Marshall DM. Enzyme activities and biological functions of snake venoms. Applied Herpetology. 2005;**2**:109-123

[20] Aguilar I, Guerrero B, Salazar AM, Giron ME, Perez JC, Sanchez EE, et al. Individual venom variability in the south American rattlesnake *Crotalus durissus* cumanensis. Toxicon. 2007;**50**:214-224

[21] Gutierrez JM, Ownby CL. Skeletal muscle degeneration induced by venom phospholipases A2: Insights into the mechanisms of local and systemic myotoxicity. Toxicon. 2003;**42**:915-931

[22] Yamazaki Y, Takani K, Atoda H, Morita T. Snake venom vascular endothelial growth factors (VEGFs) exhibit potent activity through their specific recognition of KDR (VEGF receptor 2). The Journal of Biological Chemistry. 2003;**278**:51985-51988

[23] Chippaux JP, Williams V, White J. Snake venom variability: Methods of study, results and interpretation. Toxicon. 1991;**29**:1279-1303

[24] Estevão-Costa M-I, Sanz-Soler R, Johanningmeier B, Eble JA. Snake venom components in medicine: From the symbolic rod of Asclepius to tangible medical research and application. International Journal of Biochemistry & Cell Biology. 2018;**104**:94-113. DOI: 10.1016/j.biocel.2018.09.011

[25] McCleary RJ, Kini RM. Non-enzymatic proteins from snake venoms: A gold mine of pharmacological tools and drug leads. Toxicon. 2013;**62**:56-74. DOI: 10.1016/j.toxicon.2012.09.008

[26] Vyas VK, Brahmbhatt K, Bhatt H, Parmar U. Therapeutic potential of snake venom in cancer therapy: Current perspectives. Asian Pacific Journal of Tropical Biomedicine. 2013;**3**(2):156-162. DOI: 10.1016/S2221-1691(13)60042-8

[27] Jain D, Kumar S. Snake venom: A potent anticancer agent. Asian Pacific Journal of Cancer Prevention. 2012;**13**(10):4855-4860. DOI: 10.7314/apjcp.2012.13.10.4855

[28] de Oliveira Junior NG, e Silva Cardoso MH, Franco OL. Snake venoms: Attractive antimicrobial proteinaceous compounds for therapeutic purposes. Cellular and Molecular Life Sciences. 2013;**70**(24):4645-4658. DOI: 10.1007/s00018-013-1345-x

[29] Woolf CJ. Pain: Morphine, metabolites, mambas, and mutations. The Lancet. Neurology. 2013;**12**(1):18-20. DOI: 10.1016/S1474-4422(12)70287-9

[30] Osipov A, Utkin Y. Effects of snake venom polypeptides on central nervous

system. Central Nervous System Agents in Medicinal Chemistry. 2012;**12**(4):315-328. DOI: 10.2174/187152412803760618

[31] Reptile Venom Research. Australian Reptile Park. Archived: February 2, 2010. Retrieved: December 21, 2010

[32] Boulenger GA. The Snakes of Europe, Publisher. London: Methuen; 1913

[33] Siegel AB, Zhu AX. Metabolic syndrome and hepatocellular carcinoma: Two growing epidemics with a potential link. Cancer. 2009;**115**:5651-5661

[34] Gao J, Xie L, Yang WS, Zhang W, Gao S, Wang J, et al. Risk factors of hepatocellular carcinoma–current status and perspectives. Asian Pacific Journal of Cancer Prevention. 2012;**13**:743-752

[35] Boudou-Rouquette P, Narjoz C, Golmard JL, Thomas-Schoemann A, Mir O, Taieb F, et al. Early sorafenib-induced toxicity is associated with drug exposure and UGTIA9 genetic polymorphism in patients with solid tumors: A preliminary study. PLoS One. 2012;**7**:e42875

[36] El-Magd MA, Mohamed Y, El-Shetry ES, Elsayed SA, Abo-Gazia M, Abdel-Aleem GA, et al. Melatonin maximizes the therapeutic potential of non-preconditioned MSCs in a DEN-induced rat model of HCC. Biomedicine & Pharmacotherapy. 2019;**114**:108732

[37] Shaban AM, Hammouda O, Abou Ghazala L, Raslan M, El-Magd MA. Ethyl acetate fraction of garlic (*Allium sativum*) inhibits the viability of MCF7 and HepG2 through induction of apoptosis and G2/M phase cell cycle arrest. Journal of Applied Pharmaceutical Science. 2018; **8**:142-150

[38] Mansour GH, El-Magd MA, Mahfouz DH, Abdelhamid IA, Mahamed MF, Ibrahim NS, et al. Bee venom and its active component Melittin synergistically potentiate the anticancer effect of Sorafenib against HepG2 cells. Bioorganic Chemistry, November 2021;**116**:105329

[39] Nassar MI, Elzayat EM. Anti-cancer and anti-microbial and neurological effects using wasp venom peptides agents: Review. Acta Scientific Microbiology. 2020;**3**(1):97-102

[40] Nassar MI. Wasps venom new trend for treatment of cancer, microbial and pathogenic diseases. Journal of Pharmaceutical Microbiology. 2020;**6**(2):30-31

[41] Ibrahim NM, Abd El-Monem DH, Youssef M, Ibrahim SM, Mohamed SM, Abd-Aldayem MS, et al. Bee venom drug potentiality on the macro molecules damage of the larval gut of *Hermetia Illucens* (L.), (Diptera: Stratiomyidae). Journal of the Egyptian Society of Parasitology. 2020;**50**(3):488-493

[42] Mansour GH, El-Magd MA, Mahfouz DH, Abdelhamid IA, Mohamed MF, Ibrahim NS, et al. Bee venom and its active component Melittin synergistically potentiate the anticancer effect of Sorafenib against HepG2 cells. Bioorganic Chemistry. 2021;**3**(116):105329. DOI: 10.1016/j.bioorg.2021.105329

[43] Estevão-Costa M-I, Sanz-Soler R, Johanningmeier B. Johannes A Eble. Snake venom components in medicine: From the symbolic rod of Asclepius to tangible medical research and application. The International Journal of Biochemistry & Cell Biology. 2018;**09**:011. DOI: 10.1016/j.biocel.2018.09.011

[44] Mackessy SP. Handbook of Venoms and Toxins of Reptiles. Boca Raton, FL: CRC Press/Taylor & Francis Group; 2009

[45] Bauchot R. Snakes: A Natural History. New York City, NY, USA: Sterling Publishing Co., Inc.; 1994. pp. 194-209. ISBN 978-1-4027-3181-5

[46] Condrea E, Devries A, Mager J. Hemolysis and splitting of human erythrocyte phospholipids by snake venoms. Biochimica et Biophysica Acta (BBA)—Specialized Section on Lipids and Related Subjects. 1964;**84**(1):60-73. DOI: 10.1016/0926-6542(64)90101-5

[47] Tan KK, Bay BH, Gopalakrishnakone P. L-amino acid oxidase from snake venom and its anticancer potential. Toxicon. 2018;**144**:7-13

[48] Ullah A. Structure-function studies and mechanism of action of snake venom L-amino acid oxidases. Frontiers in Pharmacology. 2020;**11**:110-110

[49] Guo C, Liu S, Dong P, Zhao D, Wang C, Tao Z, et al. Akbu-LAAO exhibits potent anti-tumor activity to HepG2 cells partially through produced H2O2 via TGF-β signal pathway. Scientific Reports. 2015;**5**:18215

[50] Abdelkafi-Koubaa Z, Aissa I, Morjen M, Kharrat N, El Ayeb M, Gargouri Y, et al. Interaction of a snake venom L-amino acid oxidase with different cell types membrane. International Journal of Biological Macromolecules. 2016;**82**:757-764

[51] Ande SR, Kommoju PR, Draxl S, Murkovic M, Macheroux P, Ghisla S, et al. Mechanisms of cell death induction by L-amino acid oxidase, a major component of ophidian venom. Apoptosis: An International Journal on Programmed Cell Death. 2006;**11**:1439-1451

[52] Burin SM, Berzoti-Coelho MG, Cominal JG, Ambrosio L, Torqueti MR, Sampaio SV, et al. The L-amino acid oxidase from *Calloselasma rhodostoma* snake venom modulates apoptomiRs expression in Bcr-Abl-positive cell lines. Toxicon. 2016;**120**:9-14

[53] Zhang H, Teng M, Niu L, Wang Y, Wang Y, Liu Q, et al. Purification, partial characterization, crystallization and structural determination of AHP-LAAO, a novel L-amino-acid oxidase with cell apoptosis-inducing activity from *Agkistrodon halys* pallas venom. Acta Crystallographica Section D: Structural Biology—Acta Crystallographica. 2004;**60**:974-977

[54] Lee ML, Fung SY, Chung I, Pailoor J, Cheah SH, Tan NH. King cobra (*Ophiophagus hannah*) venom L-amino acid oxidase induces apoptosis in PC-3 cells and suppresses PC-3 solid tumor growth in a tumor xenograft mouse model. International Journal of Medical Sciences. 2014;**11**:593-601

[55] Torii S, Yamane K, Mashima T, Haga N, Yamamoto K, Fox JW, et al. Molecular cloning and functional analysis of apoxin I, a snake venom-derived apoptosis-inducing factor with *L*-amino acid oxidase activity. Biochemistry. 2000;**39**:3197-3205

[56] Boonen A, Severens JL. The burden of illness of rheumatoid arthritis. Clinical Rheumatology. 2011;**30**(1):3-8. DOI: 10.1007/s10067-010-1634-9

[57] Grassi W, De Angelis R, Lamanna G, Cervini C. The clinical features of rheumatoid arthritis. European Journal of Radiology. 1998;**27**:S18-S24. DOI: 10.1016/S0720-048X(98)00038-2

[58] Maggie M. Potential Therapeutic Effects of Snake Venom Components on Pain Management in Rheumatoid Arthritis Patients. University Honors Theses. Paper 1075; 2021. Available from: https://doi.org/10.15760/honors.1101

[59] Heiberg T, Finset A, Uhlig T, Kvien TK. Seven year changes in health

status and priorities for improvement of health in patients with rheumatoid arthritis. Annals of the Rheumatic Diseases. 2005;**64**(2):191-195. DOI: 10.1136/ard.2004.022699

[60] Klooster PM, Veehof MM, Taal E, Riel Piet LCM, van de Laar MAFJ. Changes in priorities for improvement in patients with rheumatoid arthritis during 1 year of anti-tumour necrosis factor treatment. Annals of the Rheumatic Diseases. 2007;**66**(11):1485-1490. DOI: 10.1136/ard.2007.069765

[61] Wolfe F, Michaud K. Assessment of pain in rheumatoid arthritis: Minimal clinically significant difference, predictors, and the effect of anti-tumor necrosis factor therapy. The Journal of Rheumatology. 2007;**34**(8):1674-1683

[62] Lee YC. Effect and treatment of chronic pain in inflammatory arthritis. Current Rheumatology Reports. 2013;**15**(1):300

[63] Lee YC. Arthritis Research Introductory: Cell-Cell Adhesion Trafficking and Angiogenesis. Ann Arbor, MI: Internal Medicine—Rheumatology, University of Michigan Medical School; 2012

[64] Colmegna I, Ohata BR, Menard HA. Current understanding of rheumatoid arthritis therapy. Clinical Pharmacology & Therapeutics. 2012;**91**(4):607-620

[65] Johns Hopkins Arthritis Center. Rheumatoid Arthritis Treatment. 2018. Available from: https://www.hopkinsarthritis.org/arthritis-info/rheumatoid-arthritis/ra-treatment/

[66] Vardeh D, Naranjo JF. Peripheral and central sensitization. In: Pain Medicine. Cham: Springer; 2017. pp. 15-17. DOI: 10.1007/978-3-319-43133-8_4

[67] Cheng B, Zhou X, Zhu Q, Gong S, Qin Z, Reid P, et al. Cobratoxin inhibits pain-evoked discharge of neurons in thalamic parafascicular nucleus in rats: Involvement of cholinergic and serotonergic systems. Toxicon: Official Journal of the International Society on Toxinology. 2009;**54**:224-232. DOI: 10.1016/j.toxicon.2009.04.007

[68] Gomes A. Snake venom—An anti arthritis natural product. Al Ameen Journal of Medical Sciences. 2010;**3**(3):176

[69] Ruan Y, Yao L, Zhang B, Zhang S, Guo J. Anti-inflammatory effects of neurotoxin-Nna, a peptide separated from the venom of *Naja naja atra*. BMC Complementary and Alternative Medicine. 2013;**13**(1):1-5. DOI: 10.1186/1472-6882-13-86

[70] Zhu KZ, Liu YL, Gu JH, Qin ZH. Antinociceptive and anti-inflammatory effects of orally administrated denatured naja naja atra venom on murine rheumatoid arthritis models. Evidence-based Complementary and Alternative Medicine. 2013;**2013**(4):1-10. DOI: 10.1155/2013/616241

[71] Chen CX, Chen JY, Kou JQ, Xu YL, Wang SZ, Zhu Q, et al. Suppression of inflammation and arthritis by orally administered cardiotoxin from *Naja naja atra*. Evidence-based Complementary and Alternative Medicine. 2015;**2015**:1-12. DOI: 10.1155/2015/387094

[72] Gomes A, Datta P, Das T, Biswas AK, Gomes A. Anti arthritic and anti inflammatory activity of a cytotoxic protein NN-32 from Indian spectacle cobra (*Naja naja*) venom in male albino rats. Toxicon. 2014;**90**:106-110. DOI: 10.1016/j.toxicon.2014.07.002

[73] Liu YL, Lin HM, Zou R, Wu JC, Han R, Raymond LN, et al. Suppression of complete Freund's adjuvant-induced adjuvant arthritis by cobratoxin. Acta Pharmacologica Sinica. 2009;**30**(2):219-227. DOI: 10.1038/aps.2008.20

[74] Schett G, Coates LC, Ash ZR, Finzel S, Conaghan PG. Structural damage in rheumatoid arthritis, psoriatic arthritis, and ankylosing spondylitis: Traditional views, novel insights gained from TNF blockade, and concepts for the future. Arthritis Research & Therapy. 2011;**13**(Suppl 1):S4. DOI: 10.1186/1478-6354-13-S1-S4

[75] Zhu Q, Huang J, Wang SZ, Qin ZH, Lin F. Cobrotoxin extracted from Naja atra venom relieves arthritis symptoms through anti-inflammation and immunosuppression effects in rat arthritis models. Journal of Ethnopharmacology. 2016;**194**:1087-1095. DOI: 10.1016/j.jep.2016.11.009

[76] Park MH, Song HS, Kim KH, Son DJ, Lee SH, Yoon DY, et al. Cobrotoxin inhibits NF-κB activation and target gene expression through reaction with NF-κB signal molecules. Biochemistry. 2005;**44**(23):8326-8336. DOI: 10.1021/bi050156h

[77] Metzger, Maggie, Potential therapeutic effects of snake venom components on pain management in rheumatoid arthritis patients [University Honors Theses. Paper 1075. 2021]. DOI: 10.15760/honors.1101

[78] Vyas VK, Brahmbhatt K, Bhatt H, Parmar U. Therapeutic potential of snake venom in cancer therapy: Current perspectives. Asian Pacific Journal of Tropical Biomedicine. 2013;**3**(2):156-162. DOI: 10.1016/S2221-1691(13)60042-8

[79] Naumann GB, Silva LF, Silva L, Faria G, Richardson M, Evangelista K. Cytotoxicity and inhibition of platelet aggregation caused by an *L*-amino acid oxidase from *Bothrops leucurus* venom. Biochimica et Biophysica Acta. 2011;**1810**:683-694

[80] Ahn MY, Lee BM, Kim YS. Characterization and cytotoxicity of *L*-amino acid oxidase from the venom of king cobra (*Ophiophagus hannah*). The International Journal of Biochemistry & Cell Biology. 1997;**29**:911-919

[81] Gebrim LC, Marcussi S, Menaldo DL, De Menezes CSR, Nomizo A, Hamaguchi A. Antitumor effects of snake venom chemically modified Lys49 phospholipase A2-like BthTX-I and a synthetic peptide derived from its C-terminal region. Biologicals. 2009;**37**:222-229

[82] Das T, Bhattacharya S, Halder B, Biswas A, Gupta SD, Gomes A. Cytotoxic and antioxidant property of a purified fraction (NN-32) of Indian Naja naja venom on Ehrlich ascites carcinoma in BALB/c mice. Toxicon. 2011;**57**:1065-1072

[83] Sun LK, Yoshii Y, Hyodo A, Tsurushima H, Saito A, Harakuni T, et al. Apoptotic effect in the glioma cells induced by specific protein extracted from Okinawa habu (*Trimeresurus flavoviridis*) venom in relation to oxidative stress. Toxicology In Vitro. 2003;**17**:169-177

[84] Karthikeyan R, Karthigayan S, Sri Balasubashini M, Somasundaram ST, Balasubramanian T. Inhibition of Hep2 and HeLa cell proliferation *in vitro* and EAC tumor growth *in vivo* by *Lapemis curtus* (Shaw 1802) venom. Toxicon. 2008;**51**(157-161):50

[85] Lin KL, Su JC, Chien CM, Chuang PW, Chang LS, Lin SR. Down-regulation of the JAK2/PI3K-mediated signaling activation is involved in Taiwan cobra cardiotoxin III-induced apoptosis of human breast MDA-MB-231 cancer cells. Toxicon. 2010;**55**:1263-1273

[86] Nunes ES, Souza MA, Vaz AF, Silva TG, Aguiar JS, Batista AM. Cytotoxic effect and apoptosis induction by *Bothrops leucurus* venom lectin on tumor cell lines. Toxicon. 2012;**59**:667-671

[87] Nolte S, De Castro DD, Barea AC, Gomes J, Magalhães A, Mello Zischler LF. A lectin purified from *Bothrops jararacussu* venom, induces apoptosis in human gastric carcinoma cells accompanied by inhibition of cell adhesion and actin cytoskeleton disassembly. Toxicon. 2012;**59**:81-85

[88] Iqbal Alam M, Ojha R, Alam MA, Quasimi H. Therapeutic potential of snake venoms as antimicrobial agents. Frontiers in Drug, Chemistry and Clinical Research, Oat. 2019;**2**:3-9. DOI: 10.15761/FDCCR.1000136

[89] Reid PF. Alpha-cobratoxin as a possible therapy for multiple sclerosis: A review of the literature leading to its development for this application. Critical Reviews in Immunology. 2007;**27**:291-302

[90] Ferreira BL, Santos DO, Dos Santos AL, Rodrigues CR, de Freitas CC, et al. Comparative analysis of viperidae venoms antibacterial profile: A short communication for proteomics. Evidence-based Complementary and Alternative Medicine. 2011;**2011**:1-4

[91] San TM, Vejayan J, Shanmugan K, Ibrahim H. Screening antimicrobial activity of venoms from snakes commonly found in Malaysia. Journal of Applied Sciences. 2010;**10**:2328-2332

[92] Lee ML, Tan NH, Fung SY, Sekaran SD. Antibacterial action of a heat-stable form of L-amino acid oxidase isolated from king cobra (*Ophiophagus hannah*) venom. Comparative Biochemistry and Physiology. Toxicology & Pharmacology. 2011;**153**:237-242

[93] Samy PR, Gopalakrishnakone P, Ho B, Chow VT. Purification, characterization and bactericidal activities of basic phospholipase A2 from the venom of Agkistrodon halys (*Chinese pallas*). Biochimie. 2008;**90**:1372-1388

[94] Xie JP, Yue J, Xiong YL, Wang WY, Yu SQ. In vitro activities of small peptides from snake venom against clinical isolates of drug-resistant mycobacterium tuberculosis. International Journal of Antimicrobial Agents. 2003;**22**:172-174

[95] Nair DG, Fry BG, Alewood P, Kumar PP, Kini RM. Antimicrobial activity of omwaprin, a new member of the waprin family of snake venom proteins. The Biochemical Journal. 2007;**402**:93-104

[96] Wang Y, Hong J, Liu X, Yang H, Liu R. Snake cathelicidin from Bungarus fasciatus is a potent peptide antibiotics. PLoS One. 2008;**3**:e3217

[97] Ciscotto P, Machado de Avila RA, Coelho EA, Oliveira J, Diniz CG, et al. Antigenic, microbicidal and antiparasitic properties of an l-amino acid oxidase isolated from *Bothrops jararaca* snake venom. Toxicon. 2009;**53**:330-341

[98] Rodrigues RS, da Silva JF, Boldrini França J, Fonseca FP, Otaviano AR, et al. Structural and functional properties of Bp-LAAO, a new L-amino acid oxidase isolated from *Bothrops pauloensis* snake venom. Biochimie. 2009;**91**:490-501

[99] Samel M, Vija H, Kurvet I, Künnis-Beres K, Trummal K, et al. Interactions of PLA2-s from Vipera lebetina, Vipera berus berus and Naja naja oxiana venom with platelets, bacterial and cancer cells. Toxins (Basel). 2013;**5**:203-223

[100] Toyama MH, Toyama Dde O, Passero LF, Laurenti MD, Corbett CE, et al. Isolation of a new L-amino acid oxidase from Crotalus durissus cascavella venom. Toxicon. 2006;**47**:47-57

[101] Tõnismägi K, Samel M, Trummal K, Rönnholm G, Siigur J, et al. L-amino acid oxidase from Vipera lebetina venom: Isolation,

characterization, effects on platelets and bacteria. Toxicon. 2006;**48**:227-237

[102] Sun MZ. Biochemical, functional and structural characterization of Akbu-LAAO: A novel snake venom L-amino acid oxidase from Agkistrodon blomhoffii ussurensis. Biochimie. 2010;**92**:343-349

[103] Kitani Y, Kikuchi N, Zhang G, Ishizaki S, Shimakura K, et al. Antibacterial action of L-amino acid oxidase from the skin mucus of rockfish Sebastes schlegelii. Comparative Biochemistry and Physiology. Part B, Biochemistry & Molecular Biology. 2008;**149**:394-400

[104] Zhang H, Teng M, Niu L, Wang Y, Wang Y, et al. Purification, partial characterization, crystallization and structural determination of AHP-LAAO, a novel L-amino-acid oxidase with cell apoptosis-inducing activity from Agkistrodon halys pallas venom. Acta Crystallographica. Section D, Biological Crystallography. 2004;**60**:974-977

[105] Xu C, Ma D, Yu H, Li Z, Liang J, et al. A bactericidal homodimeric phospholipases A2 from Bungarus fasciatus venom. Peptides. 2007;**28**:969-973

[106] Oliveira DG. Structural and functional characterization of basic PLA2 isolated from Crotalus durissus terrificus venom. Journal of Protein Chemistry. 2002;**21**:161-168

[107] Bhattacharjya S, Ramamoorthy A. Multifunctional host defense peptides: Functional and mechanistic insights from NMR structures of potent antimicrobial peptides. The FEBS Journal. 2009;**276**:6465-6473

[108] Wang Y, Zhang Z, Chen L, Guang H, Li Z, et al. Cathelicidin-BF, a snake cathelicidin-derived antimicrobial peptide, could be an excellent therapeutic agent for acne vulgaris. PLoS One. 2011;**6**:e22120

[109] Xia X, Zhang L, Wang Y. The antimicrobial peptide cathelicidin-BF could be a potential therapeutic for salmonella typhimurium infection. Microbiological Research. 2015;**171**:45-51

[110] Zhao H, Gan TX, Liu XD, Jin Y, Lee WH, et al. Identification and characterization of novel reptile cathelicidins from elapid snakes. Peptides. 2008;**29**:1685-1691

[111] Zhou H, Dou J, Wang J, Chen L, Wang H, et al. The antibacterial activity of BF-30 in vitro and in infected burned rats is through interference with cytoplasmic membrane integrity. Peptides. 2011;**32**:1131-1138

Chapter 3

# Survey of Snakes Bites among Snake Endemic Communities in North Eastern Nigeria

*Mohammad Manjur Shah, Tijjani Sabiu Imam, Aisha Bala and Zainab Tukur*

## Abstract

Snake envenomation is increasingly recognized as a serious, worldwide public health concern and a neglected tropical disease of global importance especially in the North Eastern Nigeria. The scarcity of data regarding such snake fauna couple with its ability to inflict immense misery to the poorest of the population justifies the need to identify such snakes and some of the clinical features of snakebite victims in these endemic areas. Both primary and secondary data were collected during the study. Result revealed that 10 venomous snake species were reported in Gombe, Taraba and Bauchi state. The most abundant snake species is the *Echis ocellantus* (Carpet or saw scaled viper) having the highest frequency of encounter followed by the *Bitis arientans* (Puff Adder) and *Naja nigricolis* (Black Spiting Cobra). The Kaltungo General Hospital in Gombe is one of the major treatment centers in the North-Eastern Nigeria. About 2945 Human snakebite cases were reported in the Hospital in the year 2018, the highest snake envenoming were observed in October with 16.1% frequency while January has the least snakebite cases of 1.7%. The burden of snakebite envenoming in the North-Eastern Nigeria is a serious public health challenge which desperately need to be addressed.

**Keywords:** North Eastern Nigeria, snake fauna, snakebite

## 1. Introduction

Snake envenomation or exposure to the toxin from snakebite is a common worldwide occurrence and especially greatest in tropical and subtropical regions. It has a devastating impact on human health as well as the economy through treatment expenditure and loss of productivity [1, 2]. The incidence of snakebite is mostly associated with the warm regions where economic activities of the inhabitants are predominantly agriculture [3].

The incidence of snakebite is sometimes under-documented. Chippaux [4] reported that annually the total number of snake-bites might exceed 5 million with snake-bite mortality of 1,25,000 in the world. It has been reported that the highest burden of snakebite incidence is seen in the rural poor communities of tropical countries in South Asia, Southeast Asia, and sub-Saharan Africa with an estimate of over 3,14,000 bites, 7300 deaths and nearly 6000 amputations occurring from snakebites annually in Sub-Saharan Africa [5].

In Nigeria the majority of snake species that are of medical importance belong to three families viz., Viperidae (Vipers and Adder), *Elapidae* (Cobras and Mambas) and *Colubridae* (Boomslag) [6]. The saw-scaled or carpet viper (*Echis ocellatus*), Cobras (*Naja* spp.) and puff adders *(Bitisarietans)* have proved to be the most important cause of mortality and morbidity. Specifically, the *Echisocellantus* is by far the most common cause of morbidity and mortality in North-Eastern Nigeria [6]. Nigeria is known to be home to a lot of diverse snake species especially in the North Eastern part of the Savannah region with 100–150 lethality in hospitals and also overall mortality of 15.6 daily in Kaltungo [7]. Snake bite envenomation survivors live with temporary or permanent disabilities such as amputation, blindness, disfigurement, mutilation and psychological consequence from depression. The exorbitant cost of antivenom and its scarcity is another problem for poor communities. Despite all that, there is a scarcity of data regarding such snake fauna that can inflict such immense misery to the poor section of the population. The few available literatures restrict the species to three main species as of 2001. Treatment option and critical are provided by various workers [8, 9].

## 2. Materials and methods

### 2.1 Study design and sampling technique

The purposive sampling technique was used in sampling respondents in areas that have a history of snakebite incidence, which served as a key informant, courtesy calls was made to the chiefs of the snake charmers association with an introductory letter explaining the purpose of the study and how they can be of help. An interview was conducted comprising 18 professional snake charmers with good knowledge of snakes from various local governments in the North eastern States. Based on the outcome of the interview, ten (10) professional snake charmers were recruited to participate in the study for effective snake capture. Endemic areas were sampled as a study sites and primary data were collected through the administration of questionnaires (**Figure 1**).

### 2.2 Questionnaire for collecting information on the local population

The quantitative part of the study was conducted in the community whereby the households were randomly selected in all three areas. Primary data were collected through a structured questionnaire. Purposive sampling was used to select the sample size in each village. To avoid the repetition of data, one questionnaire was administered to one participant from each household. Only individuals older than 18 years with a minimum of 3 years continuous stay in the village were interviewed. Gender was considered in order to accommodate 50% of women respondents. Participation was on a voluntary basis and oral consent.

The questionnaire comprises of closed-ended questions, this technique provided valuable information on circumstances where humans encountered snakes in their daily life. The following main issues were addressed in the questionnaire: (a) frequency of encounters with snakes (b) frequency of snakebites (c) knowledge that people have on snakes and (d) views and conceptions that people have on snakes. The response after snake encounters was also investigated. Different social and economic activities that expose human beings to snakebite, as well as correlation

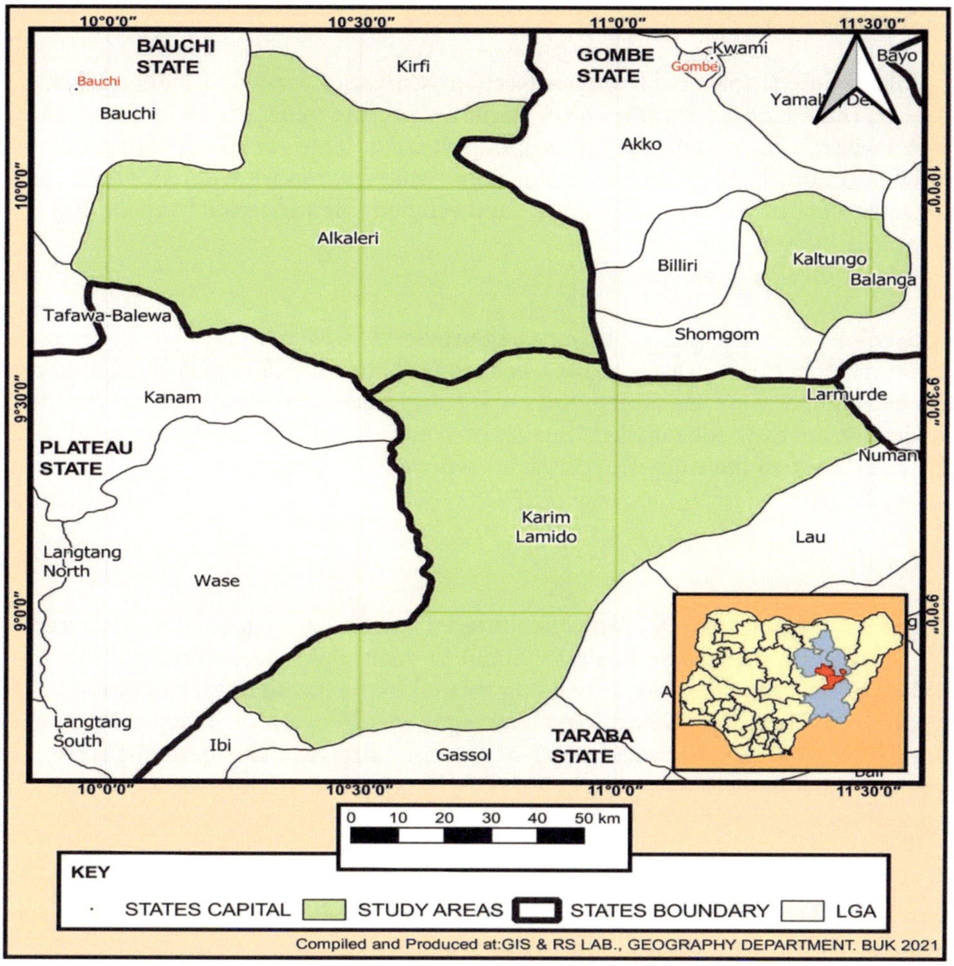


**Figure 1.**
*Map of the Snake endemic areas.*

with seasonal variation with high snakes encounters, were also studied. Applying the protocol of Kipanyula and Kimaro [10] required information is generated from the data collected.

### 2.3 Information on snakebite cases

Data on snakebites were collected at the Kaltungo General Hospital within the period of 1 year i.e. 2018. The hospital is one of the major snakebite treatment center and serves as a referral for the neighboring States as well. Furthermore, snake anti-venom is free at this center as a result of which there is huge influx of people to the center. Information was retrieved on snakebites such as the number of snakebite cases managed by the clinic, the age of the victims, as well as the type of treatment and antivenom used, etc. Snakebite victims often came with death snakes to the hospital for identification purposes and as such specimens were preserved in 4% formalin fixative medium in order to keep the snake intact with minimum artifacts. This method has been proved to be a highly efficient way of gathering large numbers of specimens.

### 2.4 Morphological data

All specimens collected from both field investigations and treatment centers were examined. Some morphometric variables such as color pattern of the snake were assessed. The quantitative phospholipidosis variable such as scale pattern, number of dorsal scale rows, ventral and sub-caudal scales were noted. These entire variables were assessed for an accurate and efficient identification purpose [11].

#### *2.4.1 Identification of the species*

Specimens were identified using a key provided by Meirte [12] and the identification crosschecked with Spawls and Branch [13] and also Chippaux [3]. Common and local names were also noted. Keys that could be used to identify up to the species level from the book entitled "Snakes of Western and Central Africa" level were also referred to in the study (https://www.whitman.edu/snakekey).

## 3. Result

In total, 10 snake species were encountered within the span of 6 months from July to December 2018 (see **Table 1**). About 45 dead snakes were retrieved from snakebite victims while they were being treated in the hospital. The rest were captured by snake charmers/catchers during field surveys. Morphological characteristics were assessed for accurate identification purposes. The following snake species were identified as shown in **Table 1** (**Figures 2–9**). The most abundant snake species is the *Echis ocellantus* having the highest frequency of encounters.

The number of human snakebites cases reported at the Kaltungo snakebite treatment center in Gombe is presented in **Table 2**. It serves as a major free referral center for all the neighboring victims of snakebite, About 2945 snakebite cases was recorded within the year 2018, the highest snake envenoming were observed in October with 16.7%frequency while January has the least snakebite cases of 1.7%.

January happened to be the month with least incident of snake bites, while highest incident was recorded within the month of July to November. However, from July to November, the snake bites incident peaked because it is the wet season which encourages the snakes to come out from their habitats and roam because the environment and the weather is convenient for them.

The age group distribution of the reported snakebite cases is presented in the (**Table 3**) below and it indicated that most snakebite victims are between the age group of 0–20 (n = 1306) and 21–40 (n = 931) while the least are reported in the elderly.

The Gender distributions of snakebite cases reported at Kaltungo General Hospital is showed in (**Table 4**), with 78% frequency of snakebite in males while 22%were reported in females.

The result in **Table 5** shows highest distribution of 36 was obtained among 21–30 years age group while the least was 2 among the oldest age groups 51–60 and 61-above years. Subject distribution according to sex was higher among male subjects (61 out of 100).Farmers happened to have higher frequency when compared with cattle rearers (44).

**Table 6** describes incident of snake bite and frequency of snake encounter by the subjects. Most of the subjects had encounter with snakes less than 10 times per month (77/100). *Echisocellantus* is the snake species mostly having encounter with the subjects (66/100). Rainy season is the season with more frequency of snake encounter and bites (68/100).

DOI: http://dx.doi.org/10.5772/intechopen.105419

| Family | Specie | Local Names | English | Frequency of encounter | Venomous/non venomous |
|---|---|---|---|---|---|
| Viperidae | *Echisocellantus* | Kububuwa/gobeda nisa | Carpet viper | 28(46) | Venomous |
| Viperidae | *Bitisarientans* | Kasa | Puff adder | 13(21) | Venomous |
| Viperidae | *Causus meculatus* | — | Night adder | 7(11) | Venomous |
| Elapidae | *Najanigricolis* | Kumurci | Black spitting cobra | 4(6.5) | Venomous |
| Elapidae | *Najakatiensis* | — | Malian cobra | 2(3.2) | Venomous |
| Elapidae | *Najanivea* | — | Cape cobra | 1(1.6) | Venomous |
| Elapidae | *Dendrospis angusticep* | — | Green cobra | 1(1.6) | Venomous |
| Elapidae | *D. polylepis* | Damatsiri/micinzinmata | Black mamba | 2(3.2) | Venomous |
| Elapidae | *Naja haje* | Gansheka | Egyptian cobra | 1(1.6) | Venomous |
| Colubridae | *Dispholidus typus* | - | Bloomslang | 1(1.6) | Venomous |
| | *Python sebae* | | Rock python | 1(1.6) | Venomous |
| | | | | 1(1.6) | Non venomous |
| | | | | 61 | |

**Table 1.**
*A list of snake species of the Alkaleri, Kaltungo and Karim Lamido North-Eastern Nigeria.*

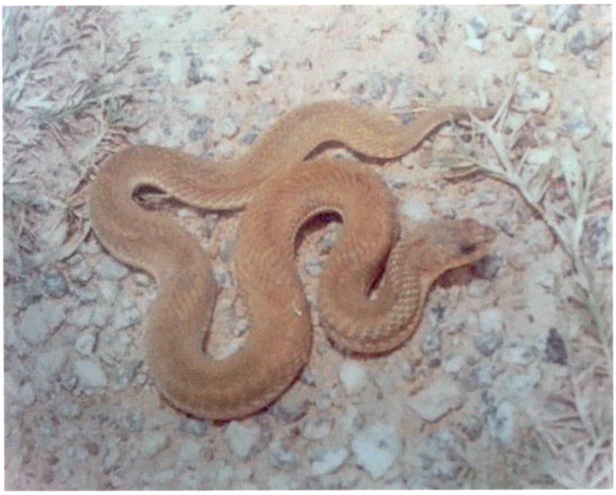

**Figure 2.**
*Cerastes cerastes (Horned viper).*

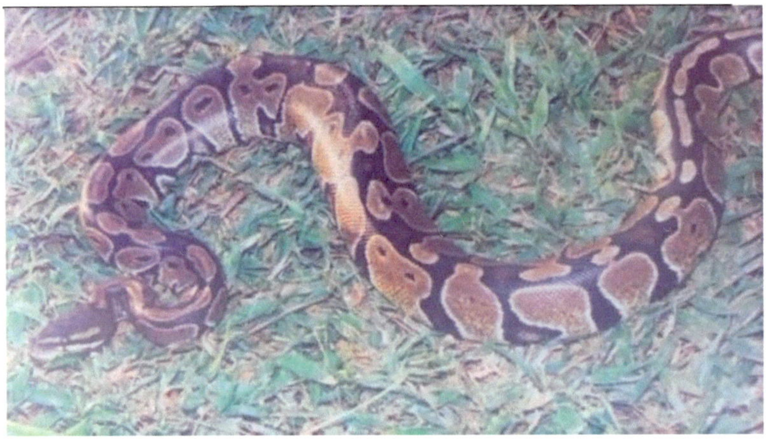

**Figure 3.**
*Pythosebae (Rock python).*

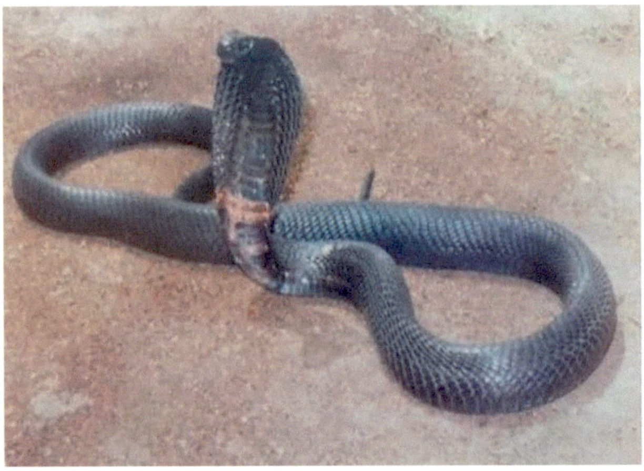

**Figure 4.**
*Naja nigricolis (Black spitting cobra).*

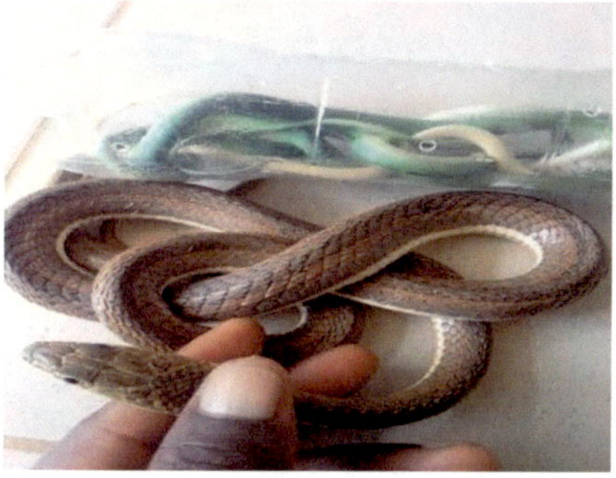

**Figure 5.**
*Dendrospis angusticep (Green cobra).*

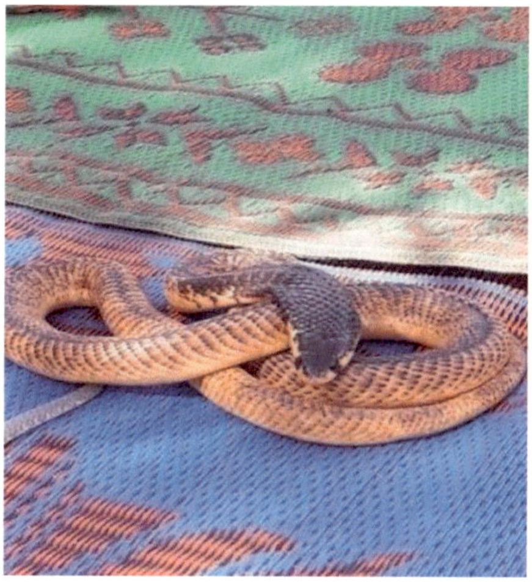

**Figure 6.**
*Naja nivea (Cape cobra).*

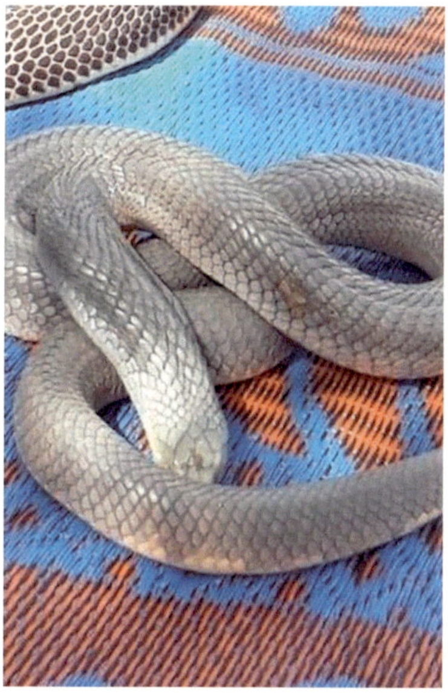

**Figure 7.**
*Dendrospis polylepis (Black cobra).*

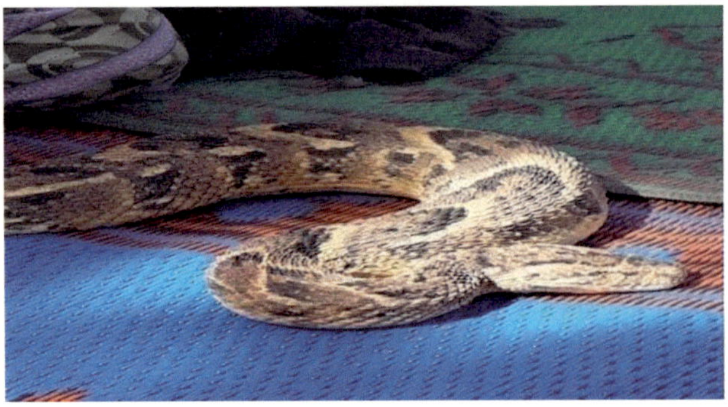

**Figure 8.**
*Bitis arientan (puff Adder).*

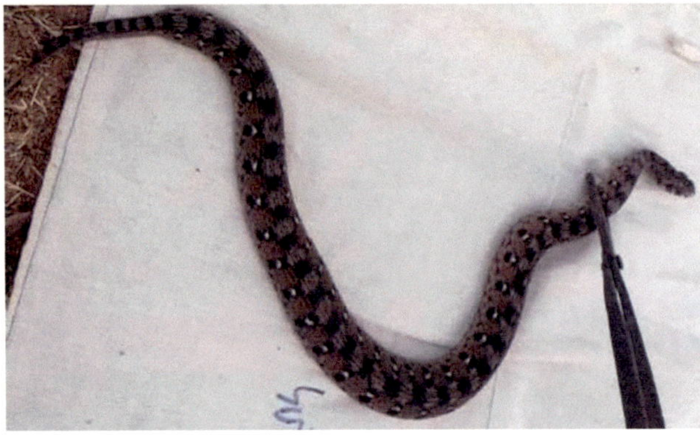

**Figure 9.**
*Echis ocellantus (Carpet viper).*

| Months | Number of snakebite | Percentage frequency (%) |
|---|---|---|
| January | 53 | 1.7 |
| February | 137 | 4.6 |
| March | 138 | 4.6 |
| April | 229 | 7.7 |
| May | 230 | 7.8 |
| June | 257 | 8.7 |
| July | 356 | 12 |
| August | 347 | 11.7 |
| September | 345 | 11.7 |
| October | 485 | 16.5 |
| November | 311 | 10.5 |
| December | 57 | 1.9 |
| Total | 2945 | 100 |

**Table 2.**
*The number of snakebite cases reported At the Kaltungo general hospital over the period of one year 2018.*

| Age group (years) | Number of snakebite | Percentage frequency (%) |
|---|---|---|
| 1–20 | 1306 | 44 |
| 21–40 | 931 | 31 |
| 41–60 | 635 | 21 |
| 61 ≥ | 73 | 2.5 |

**Table 3.**
*Age group distributions of snakebite cases reported At Kaltungo general hospital.*

| Gender | Frequency of snakebite | Percentage (%) |
|---|---|---|
| **Females** | 649 | 22 |
| **Males** | 2296 | 78 |
| **Total:** | 2, 945 | 100 |

**Table 4.**
*Gender distributions of snakebite cases reported at Kaltungo General Hospital.*

| Variable | Kaltungo (%) | Alkaleri (%) | Karim Lamido% | Total |
|---|---|---|---|---|
| Age group (yrs) | | | | |
| 18–20 | 14(15.5) | 5(5.5) | 7(7.7) | 26 |
| 21–30 | 8(8.8) | 15(15.5) | 11(12.2) | 33 |
| 31–40 | 5(5.5) | 7(7.7) | 8(8.8) | 20 |
| 41–50 | 2(2.2) | 2(2.2) | 1(1.1) | 5 |
| 51–61 | 0 | 1(1.10) | 1(1.1) | 4 |
| 61 above | 1(1.1) | 1(1.1) | 0 | 2 |
| Total | 30 | 30 | 30 | 100 |
| Sex | | | | |
| Male | 24(26.6) | 20(22.2) | 27(30) | 78.6 |
| Female | 6(6.5) | 10(11.1) | 3(3.3) | 20.9 |
| Total | 30 | 30 | 30 | 100 |
| Occupation | | | | |
| Farming | 16(18) | 21(23) | 14(15) | 56 |
| Cattle rearers | 14(15) | 9(10) | 16(17) | 42 |
| Total | 30 | 30 | 30 | 100 |

**Table 5.**
*Socio-demographic characteristics of respondent from Gombe (Kaltungo), Bauchi (Alkalarie) and Taraba (Karim Lamido).*

| Variable | | Kaltungo % | Alkaleri % | Karim Lamido% |
|---|---|---|---|---|
| Snake encountered | Few | | | |
| | Highly | 30(33) | 30(33) | 25(27.7) |
| | Moderately | 0 | 0 | 5(5.5) |
| Monthly encounter | <10 | 19(21) | 25(27.7) | 29(32) |
| | 20–30 | 10(11.1) | 5(5.5) | 1(1.1) |
| | >30 | 1(1.1) | 0 | 0 |

| Variable | | Kaltungo % | Alkaleri % | Karim Lamido% |
|---|---|---|---|---|
| Most snake spp. encountered | *Echisocellantus* | 28(31.1) | 20(22.2) | 18(20) |
| | *Bitisarientans* | 1(1.1) | 2(2.2) | 7(7.7) |
| | *Causus meculatus* | 0 | 1(1.1) | 1(1.1) |
| | *Najanigricolis* | 1(1.1) | 4(4.4) | 3(3.3) |
| | *Najakatiensis* | 0 | 1(1.1) | 1(1.1) |
| | *Najanivea* | 0 | 0 | 0 |
| | *Dendrospis angusticep* | 0 | 1(1.1) | 0 |
| | | | 1(1.1) | 0 |
| Time of the year | *D. polylepis* | 0 | 0 | 0 |
| Circumstance of | *Naja haje* | 0 | 0 | 0 |
| Bite | *Dispholidus typus* | 0 | 0 | 0 |
| Site of bite | Rainy season | 22(24.6) | 20(22.2) | 25(27.70 |
| Time of bite | Dry season | 8 | 10(11.1) | 5(5.5) |
| Snakebite treatment | Walking | 8 | 14 | 5 |
| center | Working | 22(24.6) | 16 | 25(27.7) |
| Limiting snake | Hand | 4(4.4) | 7(7.7) | 6(6.6) |
| | Leg | 26(28.8) | 22(24.6) | 23 |
| | Eye | 0 | 1 | 1(1.1) |
| | Morning | 5(5.5) | 3(3.3) | 18(20) |
| | Evening | 22(24.6) | 27(30) | 12(13.3) |
| | Night | 2(2.2) | 0 | 1(1.1) |
| | Yes | 30(33.3) | 30(33.3) | 0 |
| | No | 0 | 0 | 30(33.3) |
| | Rearing pig | 25(27.7) | 23(25.5) | 28(31.1) |
| | killing | 5(5.5) | 6(6.6) | 2(2.2) |
| | planting trees | 0 | 1(1.1) | 0 |

**Table 6.**
*Incidence of snakebite and encounter.*

## 4. Discussion

In this study 10 venomous snake species were recorded in the North Eastern State of Gombe, Taraba and Bauchi which are snake endemic communities in Nigeria. The climatic condition of the region provides an ideal environment for such savannah dwelling faunas. Similar species were also reported by previous researchers based on hospital survey records [14]. It also correlates with other studies [15] where 14 venomous snakes were reported in Nigeria [16] with *Naja nigrocolis, Naja melanoleuca, Causus maculatus* been found in Niger Delta. North Eastern Nigeria has been designated to be haven of snake by lots of researchers as it is harboring the highest population of snakes than all other parts of the country put together [15]. *Naja nigrocolis, Bitis arientans and Dendroaspis polylepis* were also found in Northern Tanzania based on herpetofauna survey conducted by Kipanyula and Kimaro [10]. Interestingly, Togo harbors the highest number of snake species in Africa based on a recent herpetofauna survey it showed that about 91 snakes species were found throughout the country among which the Nigerian *Naja nigrocolis, Bitis arientans and D. polylepis and Echis ocellantus* were also found in the savannah region of the country [17].

The most abundant snake species obtained from the study (**Table 6**) is the *Echis ocellantus* with a frequency of 66 and it was found throughout the study area, this high abundance could be a result of the vast agricultural farmland that pests such as rodents flourished in thereby inviting their counterpart snake predators. These findings are consistence with Habib [6] that reported about 95% of snakebite morbidity and mortality to be associated *Echis ocellantus.* This finding also conforms with the studies carried out by other researchers [14, 18].

During the course of this study a total number of 2945 snakebite cases have been recorded within the year 2018 only. The Kaltungo General Hospital in Gombe has been and is still a major snakebite treatment center in the Northeast and served as a major referral center for all neighboring victims of snakebite. The anti-snake venom in this hospital is totally free this could be the reason behind the increased influx of snakebite victims to the Hospital. This correlates with several studies in this region that reported an average lethality of 100–150 in hospitals and an overall mortality of 15.6 daily in Kaltungo [7, 18–20].

The highest snakebite envenoming in (**Table 2**) was reported between the months of August to October (rainy season) with the frequency of 11.5–16%, reason might be as a result of rainy season which coincided with the peak agricultural and pastoralist activities of the people. January happened to be the month with least incident of snake bites, while highest incident was recorded within the month of July to November. This discrepancy could be due to the fact that January is a Harmattan season (a very cold and dry season) which forces all cold-blooded animals (including snakes) to hide in the caves or burrows. However, from July to November, the snake bites incident peaked because it is the wet season which encourages the snakes to come out from their habitats and roam because the environment and the weather is convenient for them. Also, most of the snakes breed in this season thereby increasing their population and thus higher contact with humans. These findings are accordance with Chippaux in 2017 that reported about 74% of hospital beds have been occupied by snakebite victims, it contradicts the study [21, 22] in forest regions bites occurs almost throughout the year.

Males are bitten more often than females as shown in (**Table 3**) with reported 61 male snakebite victims and 39 females. This wide gap could be a result of males being considered as breadwinners of their homes and they are mostly engaged in farming which is considered a major source of employment. The similar results have been obtained [23]. Similarly, bites are most common in children and adolescents as having the highest snake envenomation of 1306 (44%) this is as a result of they often play with their bare hands in burrows in search of small vertebrates to supplement their diet.

Based on the outcome of the questionnaire in (**Table 6**) 100% of the respondent from Kaltungo, Alkalarie and Bambur have encountered snakes in their life to some extent and they consider their areas to harbor the highest number of snake species. The most medically important snake species in those areas are *Echis ocellantus* (Carpet viper), *Bitis arientans* (Puff adder) and *Naja nigrocolis* (Black spitting copra). This has been documented in a lot of literatures [4, 7, 19, 24, 25].

The majority of snakebites as shown in (**Table 6**) occur either in the late afternoon or early evening, times it might occur at night while the people are sleeping. In such cases, the snakes are mostly searching for food inside houses. Interestingly according to Chippaux [4] and Habib [15] reported that some species especially *Naja* spp. are mostly nocturnal as such bites by such spp. are mostly at night.

Over 77 out of 100 of the bites are located on the lower limb, especially below the knee. This is because most of the bites occur during agricultural work, hunting, or movement related to work. Bites to the hand or eye are uncommon to rare, but not exceptional, especially among farmers who work with traditional tools with short handles or in children who dig or play with their bare hands in burrows in search of small vertebrates to supplement their diet. All these increases their chances of exposure to such snakes this is also in accordance with earlier workers [4, 24, 26].

## 5. Conclusion

Snake envenomation is increasingly recognized as a serious, worldwide public health concern and a neglected tropical disease of global importance, especially in North Eastern Nigeria. In this study, 10 venomous snake species were reported in Gombe, Taraba and Bauchi States (**Figure 1**). *Echis ocellantus* was the most abundant snake in the endemic communities. Males happened to be most affected with snake bites of 2296 (77%) more than females since they are more exposed to snakes encounter at the farms than the females. Highest snake envenoming was recorded within the month of August and October (16.1%) with least occurrence in January (1.7%).

The findings of this study will be very significant in a future studies on various applied aspects.


## Author details

Mohammad Manjur Shah[1]*, Tijjani Sabiu Imam[2], Aisha Bala[2] and Zainab Tukur[2]

1 Deparment of Biological Sciences, Yusuf Maitama Sule University, Kano, Nigeria

2 Biological Sciences Department, Bayero University, Kano, Nigeria

*Address all correspondence to: mmanjurshah@gmail.com

## References

[1] Imam TS, Tukur Z, Bala AA, Ugya YA. In vitro trichomonocidal potency of Naja nigricolis and arientans snake venom. International Journal of One Health. 2021;**7**(1):2455-8931

[2] Rahman R, Faiz MA, Selim S, Rahman B, Basher A, Jones A, et al. Annual incidence of snake bite in rural Bangladesh. PLoS Neglected Tropical Diseases. 2010;**4**(10):1-6. DOI: 10.1371/journal.pntd.0000860

[3] Chippaux JP. Reviews/analyses Snake-bites: Appraisal of the global situation. Bulletin of the World Health Organization. 1998:515-524

[4] Chippaux JP. Snake bite evenomation turns again into a neglected tropical disease. Journal of Venomous Animals and Toxins Including Tropical Diseases. 2017;**23**:38

[5] Habib AG, Lamorde M, Dalhat MM, Habib ZG, Kuznik A. Cost-effectiveness of antivenoms for snakebite envenoming in Nigeria. PLoS Neglected Tropical Diseases. 2015;**9**(1):e3381. DOI: 10.1371/journal.pntd.0003381

[6] Habib AG. Public health aspects of snakebite care in West Africa: Perspectives from Nigeria. Journal of Venomous Animals and Toxins Including Tropical Diseases. 2013;**19**(1):1. DOI: 10.1186/1678-9199-19-27

[7] Hamza M, Idris MA, Maiyaki MB, Lamorde M, Chippaux JP, Warrell DA, et al. Cost-effectiveness of antivenoms for snakebite envenoming in 16 countries in West Africa. PLoS Neglected Tropical Diseases. 2016;**10**(3):1-16. DOI: 10.1371/journal.pntd.0004568

[8] Chippaux JP, Lang J, Amadi-Eddine S, Fagot P, Le Mener V. Short report: Treatment of snake evenomation by a new polyvalent antivenom composed of highly purified F(ab)2: Result of a clinical trial in Northern Cameroon. The American Journal of Tropical Medicine and Hygiene. 1999;**61**(6):1017-1018

[9] Chippaux J, White J, Habib AG. Critical care. Toxicology. 2016:1-24. DOI: 10.1007/978-3-319-20790-2_87-1

[10] Kipanyula MJ, Kimaro WH. Snakes and snakebite envenoming in Northern Tanzania: A neglected tropical health problem. Journal of Venomous Animals and Toxins Including Tropical Diseases. 2015;**21**(1):32. DOI: 10.1186/s40409-015-0033-8

[11] Chippaux JP. The impact of dracunculiasis in a sugar-cane plantation. Transactions of the Royal Society of Tropical Medicine and Hygiene. 1992;**86**:72

[12] Meirte D. Cles de determination des serpents d'Afrique. Museum Royal d'Afrique Centrale, Tervuren Belgique Annual Series Octavo Sciencebb Zoologique. 1992;**267**:1-152

[13] Spawls S, Branch B. The Dangerous Snakes of Africa. Ralph Curtis Books, Dubai: Oriental Press; 1997. p. 192

[14] Yusuf PO, Mamman M, Ajagun E, Centre BD, Muftau S. Snakes responsible for bites in North-Eastern Nigeria. Journal of Environmental Science, Toxicology and Food Technology (IOSR-JESTFT). 2013;**9**:118-121. DOI: 10.9790/2402-09921181

[15] Habib AG, Gebi UI, Onyechukwe GC. Snake bite in Nigeria. African Journal of Medical and Health Sciences. 2001;**30**(3):171-178

[16] Akani GC, Ebere N, Franco D, Eniang EA, Petrozzi F, Politano E, et al. Correlation between annual activity patterns of venomous snakes and rural

people in the Niger Delta, southern Nigeria. Journal of Venomous Animals and Toxins Including Tropical Diseases. 2013a;**19**:1-8

[17] Ohler A, Dubois A, Glitho IA. The snake fauna of Togo: Systematics, distribution and biogeography, with remarks on selected taxonomic problems the snake fauna of Togo: Systematics, distribution and biogeography, with remarks on selected taxonomic problems. 2011;**33**(3): 325-360

[18] Abubakar SB, Abubakar IS, Habib AG, Nasidi A, Durfa N, Yusuf PO, et al. Pre-clinical and preliminary dose-finding and safety studies to identify candidate antivenoms for treatment of envenoming by saw-scaled or carpet vipers (Echis ocellatus) in northern Nigeria. Toxicon. 2010;**55**(4): 719-723

[19] Akani GC, Ebere N, Franco D, Eniang E, Petrozzi F, Politano E, et al. Correlation between annual activity patterns of venomous snakes and rural people in the Niger Delta, southern Nigeria. The Journal of Venomous Animals and Toxins including Tropical Diseases. 2013b;**19**(1):2. DOI: 10.1186/1678-9199-19-2

[20] Habib G, Raza M, Saleem M. Effect of tree leaves with or without urea as a feed supplement on nutrient digestion and nitrogen balance in sheep. Animal Feed Science and Technology. 2008;**144**(3/4):335-343

[21] Segniagbeto GH, Dubois A. The snake fauna of Togo: Systematics, distribution and biogeography, with remarks on selected taxonomic problems. Zoosystems. 2011;**33**(3): 325-360. DOI: 10.5252/z2011n3a4.KEY

[22] Warrell DA. Snake bite. The Lancet. 2010;**375**:77-88. DOI: 10.1016/S0140-6736(09)61754-2

[23] Slagboom J, Kool J, Harrison RA, Casewell NR. Haemotoxic snake venoms: Their functional activity, impact on snakebite victims and pharmaceutical promise. British Journal of Haematology. 2017;**177**(6):947-959. DOI: 10.1111/bjh.14591

[24] Katibi OS, Adepoju FG, Olorunsola BO, Ernest SK, Monsudi KF. Blindness and scalp haematoma in a child following a snakebite. African Health Sciences. 2015;**15**(3):1041-1044. DOI: 10.4314/ahs.v15i3.46

[25] Strydom MA, Bester J, Mbotwe S, Pretorius E. The effect of physiological levels of South African puff adder (Bitis arietans) snake venom on blood cells: An in vitro model. Scientific Reports. 2016;**6**(October):1-8. DOI: 10.1038/srep35988

[26] de Souza TL, Magnoli FC, Dias da Silva W. Characterization of a hemorrhage-inducing component present in Bitis arietans venom. African Journal of Biotechnology. 2015;**14**(12):999-1008. DOI: 10.5897/AJB2014.14319

Section 2

# Snake Ecology

Chapter 4

# Ecology of Red-Tongue Viper (*Gloydius ussuriensis*) in Jeju Island, South Korea

*Hong-Shik Oh and Maniram Banjade*

## Abstract

Understanding the ecology of species at risk is extremely important for their conservation and management. Due to land clearing for urban expansion, agriculture, and the import of pets, several snake species including the red-tongue viper (*Gloydius ussuriensis*) on Jeju Island of South Korea, have become threatened. We studied morphology, distribution, habitat characteristics, diet, and reproduction of red-tongue viper to provide a higher understanding of species ecology. This species on average reach 242–580 mm snout-vent length and is found in a wide range of habitat from mountain forest to lowland areas. Adult snakes prey almost entirely on amphibians followed by mammals and centipedes. The mating usually takes place in spring and birth takes place in autumn. This study points out the major threats and ill-information if addressed will not only contribute to the conservation efforts but also improve the negative attitudes that people hold toward these fascinating animals. The ecological data of *G. ussuriensis* herein provides basic information which assists in designing the management technique for conservation. Similar applications may be generalized and used to other vulnerable species to detect and quantify population ecology and risks, bolstering conservation methods that can be used to optimize the efficacy of conservation measures.

**Keywords:** *Gloydius ussuriensis*, viperidae, ecology, Jeju Island, threats

## 1. Introduction

Snakes have fascinated people for millennia. They have been integrated into a variety of myths and civilizations [1]. Despite having a limbless ectothermic body, snake species have spread throughout the Earth's biomes except for the polar area. Some species may still be found within the Arctic circle (e.g., *Vipera berus*; [2]). Snakes are one of the most misunderstood and mistreated animal species [3, 4]. Snake conservation has significant hurdles due to widespread unfavorable views of snakes and a lack of awareness of their basic biology [5]. Unfortunately, we frequently know the least about the species that are the most in need of protection because of their seeming scarcity. These difficulties are most evident for vipers (Family Viperidae, ~330 species). Vipers are species with a broad range of habitats. Only a few places such as Antarctica, Australia, New Zealand, Madagascar, the Arctic Circle, and island clusters like Hawaii are free of vipers.

Vipers are among the most poisonous family of snakes. They belong to the family Viperidae. All vipers are known for their long, hollow fangs that are hinged on a highly flexible maxillary bone. Vipers are also known for their phylogenetically extensive viviparity, parental care, and ambush forager behavior [6, 7]. In a study of 1500 randomly selected reptile species, Böhm et al. [8] have discovered that vipers are much more endangered than predicted. Even though vipers make up just 9% of all snakes [9], they account for 20% of 226 snakes classified as endangered on the International Union for Conservation of Nature (IUCN) Red List [10]. Twenty viper species are classified as vulnerable, 23 as endangered, and 11 as critically endangered globally [10].

### 1.1 Snakes in South Korea

Snakes in South Korea live like in any Asian country. The location of the country is in a temperate climatic zone that provides a territory with rich flora and fauna. The country's heterogeneous landscape is represented by plains, mountains, and sea coast. Rich forests are found not only in the plains, but also in the foothills and mountainous regions which provide excellent feeding, resting, and spawning habitats for a variety of animals as well as various herpetofauna, particularly snakes. South Korea is home to 20 species of both poisonous and non-poisonous snakes (**Table 1**). Of 600 species of venomous snakes worldwide, South Korea is home to nine species [11, 12]. These venomous snakes include three pit vipers (*Gloydius brevicaudus*, *G. ussuriensis*, and *Gloydius intermedius*) belonging to Viperidae, *Rhabdophis*

| S. No | Scientific name | Common name |
|---|---|---|
| 1 | *Dinodon rufozonatum* | Red-banded snake |
| 2 | *Elaphe davidi* | David's rat snake |
| 3 | *Elaphe dione* | Steppe rat snake |
| 4 | *Elaphe schrenckii* | Korean rat snake |
| 5 | *Elaphe taeniura* | Korean beauty snake |
| 6 | *Amphiesma vibakari* | Asian keel back |
| 7 | *Hydrophis platrrus* | Yellow-bellied sea snake |
| 8 | *Hydrophis cyanocinctus* | Annulated sea snake |
| 9 | *Hydrophis melanocephalus* | Slender-necked sea snake |
| 10 | *Vipera berus* | Common viper |
| 11 | *Oocatochus rufodorsatus* | Frog-eating rat snake |
| 12 | *Hierophis spinalis* | Slender racer |
| 13 | *Pelamis platurus* | Yellow-bellied sea snake |
| 14 | *Rhabdophis tigrinus* | Tiger keelback. |
| 15 | *Sibynophis chinensis* | Black-headed snake |
| 16 | *Gloydius brevicaudus* | Short-tailed mamushi |
| 17 | *Gloydius saxatilis* | Rock mamushi |
| 18 | *Gloydius ussuriensis* | Ussuri mamushi/Red tongue viper |
| 19 | *Laticauda semifasciata* | Chinese sea snake |
| 20 | *Laticauda laticaudata* | Blue-banded sea krait |

**Table 1.**
*List of snake species in South Korea.*

*tigrinus* belonging to Colubridae, and five marine species belonging to Elapidae [13]. Red-tongue viper (*G. ussuriensis*) has the highest venom toxicity among pit vipers based on $LD_{50}$ (lethal dose that kills 50% of the population) values, followed by *G. intermedius* and *G. brevicaudus* [14]. The venom of *G. ussuriensis*, like those of other viperids, is hemotoxic, causing hemorrhages, thromboses, and severe necrosis [14]. *G. ussuriensis* and *G. brevicaudus* are the two species responsible for the majority of snakebite incidents in South Korea, particularly the former. According to large data from Korea's Health Insurance Review & Assessment Service, poisonous snake bites impact 2315–4143 patients on average each year in South Korea.

In South Korea, *G. ussuriensis* (**Figure 1**) has a wide distribution, including the mainland of South Korea and its associated islands. Jeju, the largest Island that is rich in biodiversity, is located 73 km south of the Korean Peninsula. It is a well-known habitat for this species. However, rapid urbanization and industrialization have posed a threat to this species. In the previous two decades, Jeju Island has seen significant urbanization and industrialization, undergoing a large-scale change from agricultural land to industrial land for civilization [15]. The use of heavy equipment for farming, land clearance, and road construction has caused their high mortality. Moreover, they are killed by humans despite their important roles as prey and predators in the ecosystem. These species account for a substantial proportion of middle-order predators that keep our natural ecosystem working.

However, a comprehensive understanding of its ecology and population biology is lacking. Such gaps in our understanding hinder our capacity to design effective conservation and management plans. They also prevent us from arguing that conservation is even necessary. This seems to be because there is a lack of communication between scientists due to publications written in various languages. Most publications about *G. ussuriensis* are in the Korean language, attracting little attention from researchers who write in western languages. In an attempt to bring Korean research focusing on *G. ussuriensis* to the attention of researchers worldwide, we reviewed various publications and major findings of Kim and Oh from 2014 to 2016. Effective conservation of snakes nearly always requires answers to specific questions regarding their distribution, diet, habitat requirements, and reproduction.

### 1.2 Jeju Island

Jeju Island is a typical volcanic island formed about 2 million years ago by a volcanic eruption. It is located in the most southerly portion of the Korean

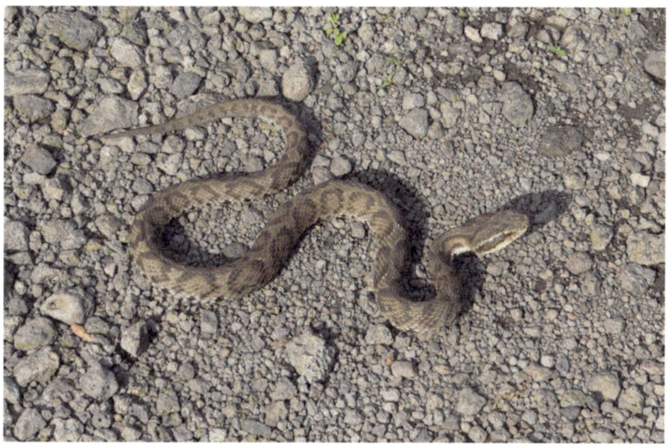

**Figure 1.**
G. ussuriensis *individual observed in Jeju Island.*

Peninsula. Its topography is smooth with an oval form extending in an east-northeast direction [16]. There is a wide range of volcanic topographies. There are about 360 small volcanoes known as "Oreum". Oreums are distributed mainly in the middle mountain zones [17] that provide retreat sites for snakes. The highest peak on the island is 1950 m above sea level. Despite its small size (1833.2 $km^2$), a total of 830.94 $km^2$ (about 45%) land area was designated as a "Biosphere Reserve" by UNESCO (United Nations Education Scientific Cultural Organization) in 2002 [18].

The climate on Jeju Island is highly seasonal with cool, dry winters and warm, wet summers. The hottest month is August (average temperature of 26.5°C) and the coldest month is January (average temperature of 6°C). It contains various habitat types ranging from evergreen broadleaf forest, deciduous forest, and coniferous forest to grassland and wetland habitats [19]. The Island supports 4764 species of land flora [19]. Vertebrate species include 43 species of mammals (including sea mammals), 418 species of birds, 7 species of amphibians, and 14 species of reptiles [20].

## 2. Description

### 2.1 Morphology

*G. ussuriensis* is a small-sized, highly venomous snake belonging to the family of Viperidae [21]. Its adults have short, moderately slender bodies not exceeding 650 mm (rarely more than 680 mm). Its tail length is 80 mm [22]. Males are generally larger than females (**Table 2**). The Head is large and often triangular because of the lateral projection of quadrate bones. Its very small eyes have typical vertical pupils with a fine bright edge. Its mouth has paired hollow fangs connected to venomous glands located behind the eye at the back upper part of the jaw. The tongue is pink or red and bifurcated. Scales are located in 21 rows on each side of the body. There are also abdominal scutes (16–66 pairs) and sub-caudal scutes (about 51 pairs).

The general ground color of the body is brown or brown of varying intensity, sometimes almost black. On the side of the body starting from the head, there is a row of elliptical or rounded dark spots with a light middle and darker edges. In the middle of the back, rings of opposite sides are often joined. The belly is yellow-gray with black marks anteriorly. In the central part, there is a combination of black and yellow-gray spots such that the snake is well camouflaged both in arboreal and terrestrial situations. Posteriorly, the belly is uniformly black. The melanistic individual from Jeju Island has been reported [24], with remarks on color variations of this species.

| **SVL (mm)** | **Population** | | |
|---|---|---|---|
| | **Male (n = 61)** | **Female (n = 99)** | **SSD (Sexual size dimorphism)** |
| Mean | 434.5 | 422.0 | |
| SD | 51.7 | 46.7 | −0.03 |
| Range | 296–580 | 242–532 | |
| | | | Kim and Oh [23] |

**Table 2.**
*Snout-vent length (SVL) comparison between male and female of* G. ussuriensis *in Jeju Island.*

## 3. Life history

### 3.1 Distribution

*G. ussuriensis* is a species of a venomous snake having limited distribution worldwide. Currently, the known range of this species cover the following regions: Russian Far East, northwards to the lower Amur River, westwards to the Argun River, eastwards limited to the coast of the Sea of Japan and Tatarskiy Strait, the Korean peninsula, and northeastern China [21, 25]. In Korean Peninsula, it is commonly found in mainland South Korea, Jeju Island, and its associated islets. In Jeju Island, its distribution is homogenous (**Figure 2**) and it is one of the most commonly encountered snakes. In Jeju Island, it utilizes various habitats ranging from mountain forests to low altitude areas containing swamps and marshes [26, 27]. They are frequented more open microhabitats that had rocks or fallen logs that served as a refuge or basking spots. Agricultural land, grasslands, and freshwater streams are the areas of most frequent records. More commonly they were recorded from wetland sites adjacent to forested habitats as; Dongbaekdongsan, Muljangori, Mulyeongari, and Sumeunmulbaengdui wetland areas. Being hygrophilous, it is not uncommon on the sea. It is also recorded at an altitude up to 1947 m. However, until recently no information is available about population size.

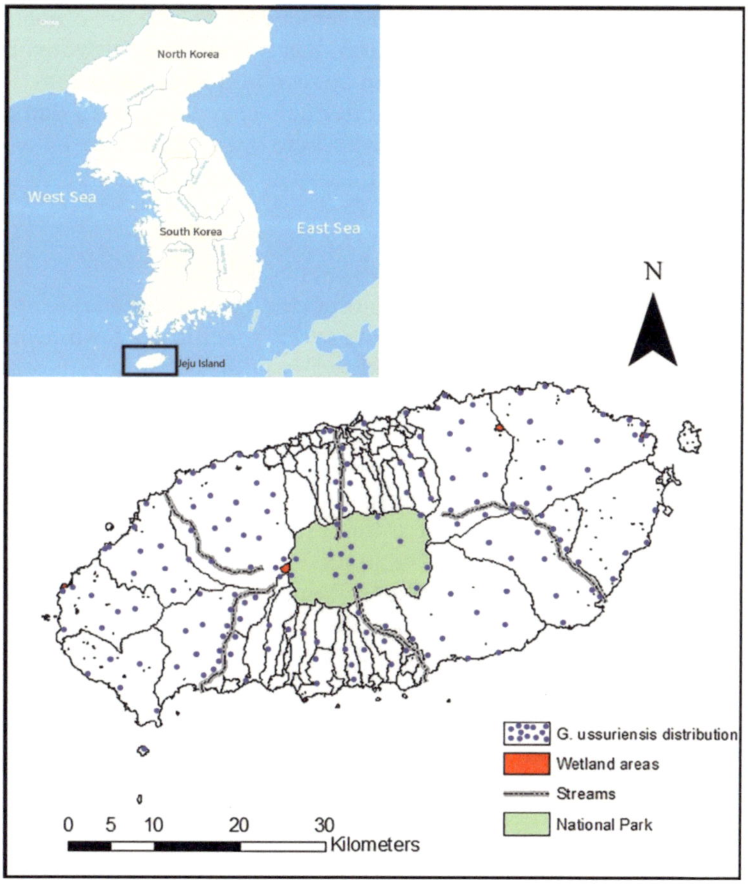


**Figure 2.**
*Distribution of* G. ussuriensis *in Jeju Island.*

### 3.2 Habit and habitat

Each species has its own unique behavior. Some spend most of the day foraging for food or basking in the sun, while others are most active at dusk and dawn or during the night. *G. ussuriensis* has plasticity in its diet, which allows this species to spread widely and survive in various landscape zones. Prey is identified by heat, followed by a sudden and rapid attack and bite. Basking in the sun is a common daytime activity in early summer. Hibernation begins from October to the middle of May of the following year. Each individual has its own hunting territory, beyond which it does not go. *G. ussuriensis* generally engages in limited movements. They may remain for long period in relatively small areas of approximately 64 $m^2$ [28], where they can be repeatedly observed. They shed their skin from time to time during molting. Bites are excruciatingly painful, producing internal organ hemorrhages as well as bleeding at bite sites.

Most animals have their preferred habitats [29, 30], which may be influenced by species-specific temporal and spatial constraints. Vipers can live in different ecosystems including woodlands, forests, rocky areas, coasts, wetlands, swamps, mountainous regions, scrubs, and others. Habitat is an essential part of their survival and life history because it allows snakes to protect themselves from predators and it can be used for hibernation, breeding ground, and ambush. They can take refuge in burrows of rodents, among rocky slopes, boggy vegetation, and dense bushes. In Russia, *G. ussuriensis* usually adheres to forest edges, rocky taluses, abandoned settlements, ruins of old houses, and cemeteries. It is frequently observed on the coast of the Sea of Japan. In Jeju Island, it is common in cultivated land, low mountain areas, and forest areas. It can be seen hiding under stones. It is often found along banks of water bodies, dried-out ditches, and low-lying damp areas that provide more humidity. As a rule, it adheres to open space covered with grass or shrubs required for successful hibernation.

### 3.3 Diet

Every snake is zoophagous (consuming other creatures). All snakes are carnivorous. They eat animals, not vegetables. Some prefer specific prey, while others will eat just about everything they can grab and swallow. Snakes hunt different prey items, including rats, mice, rabbits, frogs, insects, lizards, other snakes, birds, bats, squirrels, and so on.

The diet of *G. ussuriensis* in its distribution range is not well documented. It has been stated that this species feeds primarily on frogs and other amphibians. They also feed on small mammals and other animals [31]. Thus, the diet of *G. ussuriensis* is typically broad. Kim and Oh [23] have studied prey items of *G. ussuriensis* in Jeju Island through manual palpation methods (**Figure 3**). Through the analysis of 177 individuals from 46 locations, a variety of prey items ranging from centipedes to amphibians, reptiles, and mammals were observed (**Table 3**). Among these prey, amphibians had the highest frequency of occurrence (55.2%), followed by mammals (20.7%), centipedes (13.8%), and reptiles (10.3%). The highest occurrence of the amphibian diet of *G. ussuriensis* is related to a higher abundance of herpetofauna at swampy (wetland) areas as good habitats of *G. ussuriensis* whose subsequent mimicry can kill the prey. The choice of prey differs in response to local and geographical variation in prey availability or abundance. At Gapado Island (Islets of Jeju Island, located 5.5 km off the Jeju coast), where prey items of *G. ussuriensis* were limited only to centipedes and lizards [23]. They concluded that the shift in diet was related to the lower density of favorable prey items.

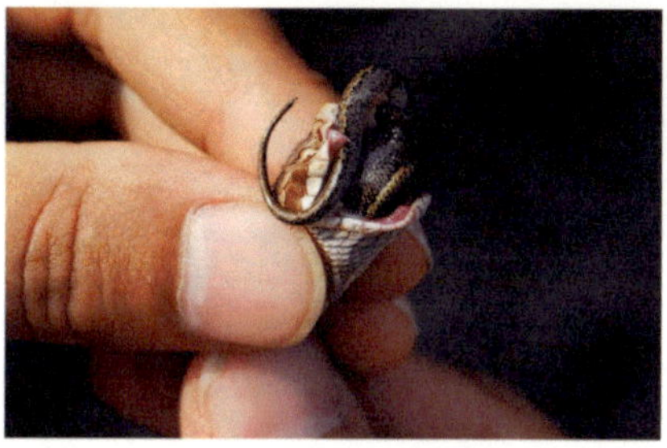

**Figure 3.**
*Prey detection of* G. ussuriensis *through manual palpation method.*

| Preys | | Number | Remarks |
|---|---|---|---|
| **Sorts** | **Scientific name** | | |
| Centipede | *Scolopendra subspinipes mutilans* | 4 | |
| | *Hynobius quelpaertensis* | 2 | |
| | *Hyla japonica* | 9 | |
| Amphibians | *Kaloula borealis* | 2 | |
| | *Rana dybowskii* | 1 | |
| | *Rana nigromaculata* | 2 | |
| | *Scincella vandenburghi* | 1 | |
| Reptiles | *Amphiesma vibakari* | 1 | |
| | *Colubridae* sp. | 1 | Skin of snakes |
| | *Crosidura shantungensis* | 1 | |
| Mammals | *Sorex caecutiens hallamontanus* | 1 | |
| | *Apodemus chejuensis* | 2 | |
| | *Deomyinae* sp. | 2 | Fur of rodent |

**Table 3.**
*Prey items of* G. ussuriensis *identified through manual palpation in Jeju Island.*

Head size and shape are not static, and however, most snake species have shown substantial flexibility in head shape [32, 33]. In a wide range of snakes, head form is surprisingly varied and has been hypothesized to be adaptive, with relative head width, in particular, is connected to the maximum prey size that may be eaten [34]. In general, larger snakes eat larger prey whereas smaller consumed smaller prey. In Jeju Island, a positive correlation was found between the size of the head of *G. ussuriensis* and the diameters of prey items [23].

### 3.4 Reproduction

Reproductive behaviors and rates vary drastically based on the species. Reproduction in snakes is controlled by the natural cycle of ambient warmth and cold [35] and red tongue vipers are no exception. Seasonal changes in light and rainfall, which impact food availability, might potentially play a role in reproduction for these ectotherms. Reproduction is dioecious. Mating takes place in April and May. The mating strategy of *G. ussurisensis* is not well documented yet but incidences of 2–3 males mating with a single female have been frequently observed (**Figure 4**).

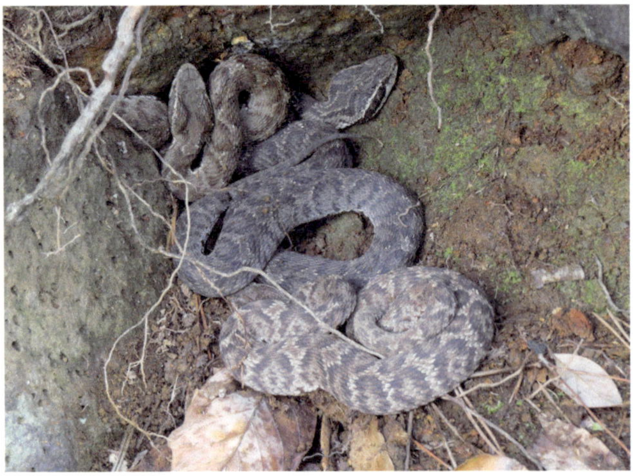

**Figure 4.**
*The group mating of* G. ussuriensis *in Jeju Island. Two male and one female participating in group mating.*

However, one incidence of multiple males competing for a single female (forming mating ball) was observed within Jeju Island (personal communication). Like other members of the viper family, *G. ussuriensis* is ovoviviparous. They retain eggs inside their bodies until they hatch and give "live" birth.

Much like other snake species, [36] red tongue viper reproduce annually. In Jeju Island, seasonal cycles based on size and histological examination of testes and follicles in ovaries have been reported by Kim and Oh [23]. The change in the monthly average value of the Testis Index (TI) was large between June and July. It was relatively stable between July and August, while it was the largest between August and early September (**Figure 5**). The average length of the largest follicle in a female's ovary was at its largest in May and smallest in June (**Figure 6**). After intensive vitellogenesis in May, ovulation and fertilization seem to occur since June. Most births occur between the end of August and September when females give birth to 2–10 offspring in one brood.

Newborn babies completely repeat the color of their parents. With the analysis of 146 newborns, the mean weight of neonates was 4.3 ± 0.7 g (range, 1.1 g–6.6 g) and the mean length (NS) of neonates was 174.3 ± 12.6 mm (range, 110–203 mm). They reach sexual maturity at a body length of 400 mm, possibly after the second or third hibernation. Before hibernation, newborn snakes have time to molt 5–6

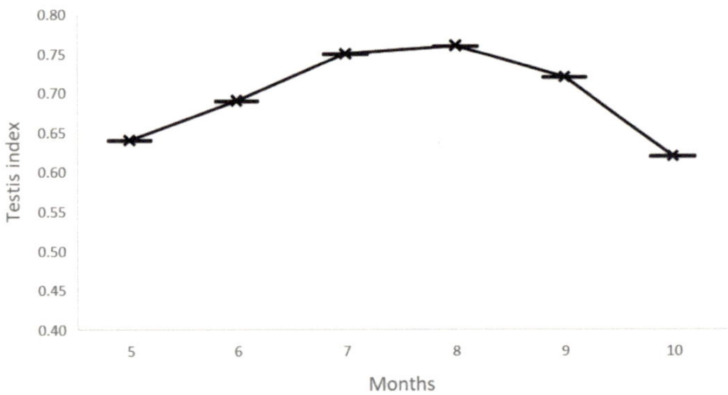


**Figure 5.**
*Monthly pattern of male testis index. Cross line represent means and horizontal lines represent standard deviation.*

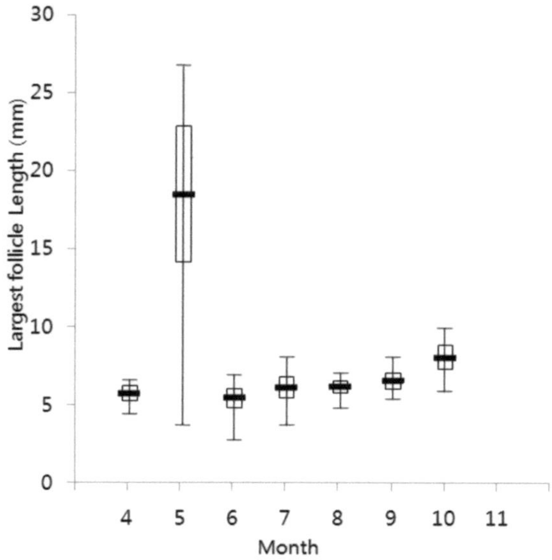


**Figure 6.**
*Annual pattern of ovarian largest follicle length in female* G. ussuriensis *in Jeju Island. Horizontal thick lines represent means and horizontal thin lines and vertical bars represent standard deviation and ranges.*

times. The first molt occurs after 6–7 h and the second molt occurs after 2–3 days. At first, newborns feed on insects and invertebrates. Later, they switch to normal food. Life expectancy on average ranges from 9 years to 15 years. In captivity, this may increase.

Adult females of many snake species breed on a less-than-annual basis, indicating the requirement of a long foraging period to accumulate sufficient reserve for offspring production [37]. *G. ussuriensis* females have a one-year breeding cycle [23]. According to indirect data, in the north of Primorsky and the Khabarovsk Territory in Russia, this species may have a two-year breeding cycle. Depending on factors such as prey densities and favorable weather conditions, some degree of synchrony is observed during clutch or litter production by females within a population.

### 3.5 Natural predators and competitors

*G. ussuriensis* members, particularly young ones, have someone to fear. They are frequently attacked by birds of prey (hawk, white-tailed eagle, and black kite), large-billed crow and jay, and predatory mammals (badger, Siberian weasel). Competition from other vipers does not seem to be occurring in Jeju Island. In many parts of the world, humans hunt vipers for food [38]. The genus Gloydius, has long been known for its medicinal value in Asia. Dried *G. ussuriensis* meat is eaten for medical treatment by inhabitants of Japan and Korea. Thus, hunting for them has made people their main enemy.

## 4. Threat

### 4.1 Habitat loss and fragmentation

The most serious risks to biodiversity are habitat loss and fragmentation. It is reasonable to believe that habitat loss and fragmentation will be the most serious dangers to snake populations worldwide [39, 40]. Where the natural forest is destroyed and replaced with intensive agriculture, coniferous plantations, or urban development, *G. ussuriensis* faces a particularly serious threat. Such changes will definitely have a detrimental effect on the prey abundance of snake species, decreasing predators' chances of long-term survival [41].

As vehicle ownership and traffic levels increase, many new roads are being built everywhere in Jeju Island, with a greater proportion of them being broad, fast highways. Snakes usually travel a certain distance in search of a mate and seek nesting sites, which force them to cross roadways. As a result, many individuals are killed on the roads. Some others interact with threats such as humans, farm equipment, vehicles, and pets (dogs and cats), which put *G. ussuriensis* populations at serious risk.

### 4.2 Introduction of invasive species

Invasive species frequently have immediate and widespread detrimental consequences for populations, natural groups, and biodiversity [42]. The impact of invasive alien species on native snakes species in the world has been recorded, including the introduction of Cane Toad (*Thinella marina*) in Australia [43], Indian Mangoose (*Herpestes javanicus*) in some Antillean Islands [44], and three species of fire ants (*Solenopsis invicta, S.geminata,* and *Wasmannia auropunctata*) in Africa and New-Zealand [45].

In 2017, a red fire ant (*S. invicta*) was discovered in South Korea. Since then, it has subsequently spread to various states within the country [46]. This species is of high concern because it has caused severe damage to many aspects of human life and wildlife [47] due to its aggressiveness and toxicity [48, 49]. Quantitative evaluation of climate suitability of the invasive red fire ant suggests that this ant has a high possibility of settlement after its introduction in Jeju Island [50]. Invasive red fire ants have the potential to harm *G. ussuriensis* indirectly through their negative effects on their prey and directly by predation facilitated by their potent stings.

### 4.3 Human persecution

The persecution of snakes by humans is widespread, especially among venomous snakes. Many snakes are killed regardless of whether they are venomous because people tend to have an irrational fear of these creatures. *G. ussueriensis* is often intentionally killed by hikers and hunters, although such an act is considered illegal. Building new roads can bring more people to formerly inaccessible places, increasing the danger of snakes being killed as a result of misinformation. Even experienced field biologists have limited knowledge of this snake's behavior and biology. It is difficult to establish a positive public perception of poisonous snakes. However, an adequate legislative framework can alleviate such issues. It is essential to educate people about the importance of snakes to modify their attitudes regarding venomous snakes.

## 5. Conclusion

*G. ussuriensis* is the most widespread species in Jeju Island and has suffered greatly, due to habitat loss, fragmentation, and increased mortality from roads and human persecution. The ecology of *G. ussuriensis* in Jeju Island was studied which aids in understanding the general biology of the species. *G. ussuriensis* is the small-sized, highly venomous viperidae having widespread distribution within Jeju Island.

Through the manual palpation method, *G. ussuriensis* was identified in consuming amphibian, centipede, reptiles, and mammals. Being dioecious, mating takes place in April and May and gives birth to live young's toward the end of August and September. A complete understanding of ecology could help in implementing the conservation and management plans. Increasing people's knowledge and understanding about snake and snakebite treatment and prevention through educational interventions like snake parks and snake museums is a low-cost method to promote a snake-friendly mindset.

Here, we attempt to provide useful knowledge to locals, scientists, and conservation agencies. Because this field is in its infancy, we are forced to rely heavily on results published in other languages, personal communication, and results of unpublished experiments. We believe that successful initiatives, even if limited in their impact are informative and might well prove broadly applicable for snake conservation.

## Acknowledgements

This research was supported by the Basic Science Research Program through the National Research Foundation of Korea (NRF) funded by the Ministry of Education (2019R1A6A1A10072987).

## Appendices and nomenclature

| | |
|---|---|
| IUCN | International Union for Conservation of Nature |
| UNESCO | United Nations Education Scientific Cultural Organization |

## Author details

Hong-Shik Oh[1]* and Maniram Banjade[2]

1 Interdisciplinary Graduate Programme in Advance Convergence Technology and Science, Faculty of Science Education, Jeju National University, Jeju, South Korea

2 Practical Translational Research Center, Jeju National University, Jeju-Si, South Korea

*Address all correspondence to: sciedu@jejunu.ac.kr

## References


[1] Whitaker Z. The indian magazine book. In: Snakeman, editor. The Story of Naturalist. 1989. p. 185

[2] Carlsson M. Phylogeography of the Adder, *Vipera berus*. Ph.D. dissertation, Acta Universitatis Upsaliensis; 2003

[3] Beaupre SJ, Duvall DJ. Integrative biology of rattlesnakes. Contributions to Biology and evolution. Bioscience. 1998;**48**:531-538

[4] Seigel R, Collins J, Novak SS. Snakes: Ecology and Evolutionary Biology. London: Macmillan; 1987. p. 529

[5] Burghardt G. Combating ophiophobia: Origins, treatment, education and conservation tools. In: Mullin SJ, Seigel RA, editors. Snakes: Ecology and Conservation. Ithaca, NY: Cornell University Press; 2009

[6] Fenwick AM, Greene HW, Parkinson CL. The serpent and the egg: Unidirectional evolution of reproductive mode in vipers? Journal of Zoological Systematics and Evolutionary Research. 2011;**44**:59-66

[7] Moon BR, Penning DA, Segall M, et al. Feeding in Snakes: Form, function, and evolution of the feeding system. In: feeding in vertebrate. Cham: Springer; 2019. pp. 527-574

[8] Bohm M, Collen B, Baillie JE, et al. The conservation status of the world' s reptiles. Biological Conservation. 2013;**157**:372-385

[9] Uetz P, Hosek J. The Reptile Database. 2015. Available from: http://www.reptile-database.org/ [Accessed: October 30, 2021]

[10] IUCN. Red List of Threatened Species, Version 2015-4. 2015. Available from: https://www.iucnredlist.org/

[11] Orlov NL, Barabanov A. Analysis of nomenclature, classification, and distribution of the *Agkistrodon halys—Agkistrodon intermedius* complexes: A critical review. Russian Journal of Herpetology. 1999;**6**:167-192

[12] Lee J, Jang H, Seo J. Ecological Guidebook of Herpetofauna in Korea. National Institute of Environmental Research. 2012. Available from: https://www.nier.go.kr/NIER/eng/index.do

[13] Shin Y, Jang Y, Borzée A. Snakebite envenomings in the Republic of Korea from the 1970s to the 2020s: A review. Toxicon. 2021;**196**:8-18

[14] Yoo C, Kim Y, Park M, et al. Determination of venom toxicity and standardization of venom and antivenin of Korean Agkistrodon spp. Korean Journal of Veterinary Public Health. 1999;**23**:135-142

[15] Hong HJ, Kim CK, Lee HW, et al. Conservation, restoration and sustanable use of biodiversity based on habitat quality monitoring: A case study on Jeju Island, South Korea (1989-2019). Land. 2021;**10**:1-15

[16] Banjade M, Han S, Jeong Y, et al. Long-term trends of bird community at Dongbaekdongsan and 1100-highland wetland of Jeju Island, South Korea. Korean Journal of Ornithology. 2019;**26**:54-61

[17] Nam H, Kim E, Choi C, et al. Avifauna of gungdae oreum and its seasonal changes in the Jeju Eastern Oreum group in Jeju Island, Korea. Journal of Asia-Pacific Biodiversity. 2019;**12**:515-521

[18] JSSGP. Periodic Review for Jeju Island Biosphere Reserve Submitted to UNESCO. 2012. Available from: https://en.unesco.org/biosphere/aspac/jeju-island

[19] MoE (Ministry of Environment, South Korea). ECOREA—An Environmental Review. 2011. Available from: https://wedocs.unep.org/handle/20.500.11822/9046?show=full

[20] Jo YS, Kim TW, Choi BJ, et al. Current status of terrestrial mammals on Jeju Island. Journal of Species Research. 2012;**1**:249-256

[21] Zhao E. Crotalinae. In: Zhao EM, Huang MH, Zong Y, editors. Fauna Sinica, Reptilia. Beijing: Science Press; 1998

[22] Emelianov A. Snakes of the far eastern district. Memoirs of the Vladivostok Section of the Russian State Geographical Society. 1929;**3**:3-208

[23] Kim B, Oh H. Food use of the red-tongue viper snake (*Gloydius ussuriensis*). Korean Journal of Environment and Ecology. 2014;**28**:657-663

[24] Shin Y, Borzee A. Melanism in the Ussuri Pitviper (*Gloydius ussuriensis*) from the Republic of Korea, with remarks on color variations. Jordan Journal of Natural History. 2020;**7**:60-63

[25] Gumprecht A, Tillack F, Orlov N, et al. Asian Pitvipers. Berlin: Geitje Books; 2004. pp. 1-368

[26] Do MS, Yoo JC. Distribution pattern according to altitude and habitat type of the red-tongue viper snake (*Gloydius ussuriensis*) in the Cheon-ma mountain. Journal of Wetland Ecology. 2014;**16**:193-204

[27] Kim BS. A study on the ecology of the Ussuri Mamushi (*Gloydius ussuriensis*) from Jeju Island, South Korea. Ph.D. dissertation, Jeju National University; 2011. p. 86

[28] Kim B, Oh H. Movement and home range of the red-tongued viper snake (*Gloydius ussuriensis*) inhabiting gapado. Korean Journal of Environment and Ecology. 2015;**29**:192-199

[29] Brown JH. Mammals on mountainsides: Elevational patterns of diversity. Wiley. 2001;**10**:101-109

[30] Martinez-Freiria F, Sillero N, Lizana M, et al. GIS-based niche models identify environmental correlates sustaining a contact zone between three species of European vipers. Diversity and Distribution. 2008;**14**:452-461

[31] Orlov N, Schuett G, Barabanov A. Biology of the Vipers. Eagle Mountain, Utah: Eagle Mountain Publishing; 2002. pp. 345-360

[32] Aubret F, Shine R, Bonnet X. Evolutionary biology: Adaptive developmental plasticity in snakes. Nature. 2004;**431**:261-262

[33] Smith MT. Induction of phenotypic plasticity in rattlesnake trophic morphology by diet manipulation. Journal of Morphology. 2014;**275**:1339-1348

[34] Vincent SE, Dang PD, Herrel A, et al. Morphological integration and adaptation in the snake feeding system: A comparative phylogenetic study. European Society for Evolutionary Biology. 2006;**19**:1545-1554

[35] Duvall D. Environmental control of reptilian reproductive cycles. Biology of Reptiles. 1982;**13**:201-231

[36] Krohmer RW. The male red-sided garter snake (*Thamnophis sirtalis parietalis*): Reproductive pattern and behavior. ILAR Journal. 2004;**45**:65-74

[37] Bonnet X, Lourdais O, Shine R, et al. Reproduction in a typical capital breeder: Costs, currencies and complications in the viper. Ecology. 2002;**83**:2124-2135

[38] Klemens M, Thorbjarnarson J. Reptiles as a food resource. Biodiversity and Conservation. 1995;**4**:281-298

[39] Wilcove DS, Rothstein D, Dubow J, et al. Quantifying threats to imperiled species in the United States. Bioscience. 1998;**48**:607-615

[40] Gibbons JW, Scott DE, Ryan TJ, et al. The global decline of reptiles, deja vu amphibians. Bioscience. 2000;**50**:653-666

[41] Brown GP, Ujvari B, Madsen T, et al. Invader impact clarifies the roles of top-down and bottom-up effects on tropical snake populations. Functional Ecology. 2013;**27**:351-361

[42] Sakai AK, Allendorf FW, Holt JS, et al. The population biology of invasive species. Annual Review of Ecology and Systematics. 2001;**32**:305-332. DOI: 10.1146/annurev.ecolsys.32.081501.114037

[43] Phillips BL, Brown GP, Shine R. Assessing the potential impact of cane toads on Australian snakes. Conservation Biology. 2003;**17**:1738-1747

[44] Henderson RW. Lesser Antillean snake faunas: Distribution, ecology, and conservation concerns. Oryx. 2009;**38**:311-320

[45] Holway DA, Lach L, Suarez AV, et al. The causes and consequences of ant invasions. Annual Reveiw Ecology, Evolution and Systematics. 2002;**33**:181-233

[46] Lyu DP, Lee HS. The red imported fire ant, solenopsis invicta buren (hymenoptera: formicidae: myrmicinae) discovered in Busan sea port, Korea. Korean Journal of Applied Entomology. 2017;**56**:437-438

[47] Vinson B. Invasion of the red imported fire ant (hymenoptera: formicidae): Spread, biology and impact. American Entomology. 1997;**43**:23-39

[48] Jemal A, Hugh-jones M. A review of the red imported fire ant (*Solenopsis invicta Buren*) and its impacts on plant, animal, and human health. Preventive Veterinary Medicine. 1993;**17**:19-32

[49] Solley GO, Vanderwoude C, Knight GK. Anaphylaxis due to red imported fire ant sting. The Medical Journal of Australia. 2002;**176**:521-523

[50] Byeon D, Lee J, Lee H, et al. Prediction of spatiotemporal invasive risk by the red imported fire ant (hymenoptera: formicidae) in South Korea. Agronomy. 2020;**10**:1-15

Chapter 5

# Comparative Ecology of Two Species of Semiaquatic Snakes in Southeastern North America

*Jeffrey D. Camper*

## Abstract

The banded water snake (*Nerodia fasciata fasciata*) and the Eastern cottonmouth (*Agkistrodon piscivorus piscivorus*) were the focal species in a long-term mark and recapture study in the upper coastal plain of South Carolina, USA. Recapture rates were low for both species. Female *N. fasciata* were significantly larger than males. Male *A. piscivorus* were larger than females but not significantly. Age structure and sex ratios were determined for these populations. Recapture latency was greater for *A. piscivorus* than for *N. fasciata*. There was little dietary niche overlap between these two species. *Nerodia fasciata* ingested significantly more fish headfirst and more amphibians tail first. Growth rates were also calculated for both species. Litter size, offspring size, relative clutch mass and parturition dates were determined for *N. fasciata*.

**Keywords:** banded water snake, Eastern cottonmouth, reproduction, food habits, population ecology, sexual dimorphism

## 1. Introduction

Certain aspects of the life history of an organism can have important fitness consequences [1]. Snakes have lagged behind other groups of vertebrates in the understanding of life history traits due to difficulties in detection and sampling [2]. Successful reproduction is the primary measure of fitness but life history parameters such as foraging success, thermoregulation and habitat choice are important to survival and therefore a prerequisite to fitness increases [3, 4]. In an attempt to elucidate the importance of these ecological factors I studied two semiaquatic snake species on the coastal plain of southeastern North America.

The banded water snake (*Nerodia fasciata*) is a moderate sized (to 1524 mm total length) heavy bodied snake with a dorsal color pattern of brown to reddish-brown bands with grayish to brown pigment between the bands [5] (**Figure 1**). The labial scales bear dark bars at their margins and a dark stripe runs from the eye to the angle of the jaw. Larger specimens frequently lose much of the banding and are uniformly brown. This species occurs throughout the coastal plain of southeastern North America from the state of North Carolina south to Florida and west to Texas [6]. It can be found in almost any body of fresh water including streams, rivers, lakes, ponds, marshes, sloughs, canals and swamps. Life history data for this species has been summarized by [5, 6].

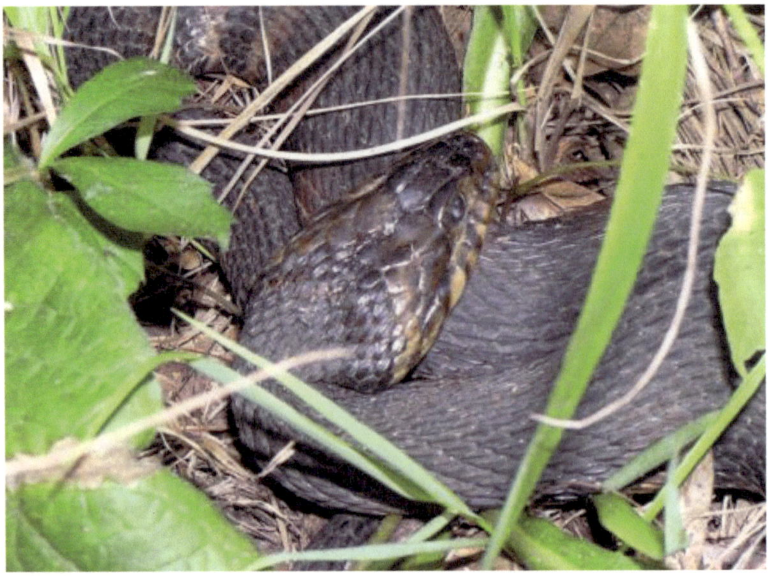

**Figure 1.**
*Adult female banded water snake (Nerodia fasciata fasciata) from the study site. Note faint bands in upper left part of photograph.*

The cottonmouth or water moccasin (*Agkistrodon piscivorus*) is a large (to 1890 mm total length) pitviper with a thick brown stripe on the side of the head that runs through the eye to the angle of the jaw (**Figure 2**). Pale lines both above and below border this stripe. The large triangular shaped head is distinctly wider than the neck and the pupil is vertically elliptical. The dorsal color pattern consists of wide dark brown bands with lighter centers that alternate with a lighter brown ground color. Many larger specimens have the banding pattern obscured and appear a uniform dark brown. The inside of the mouth is lined with white tissue and is used

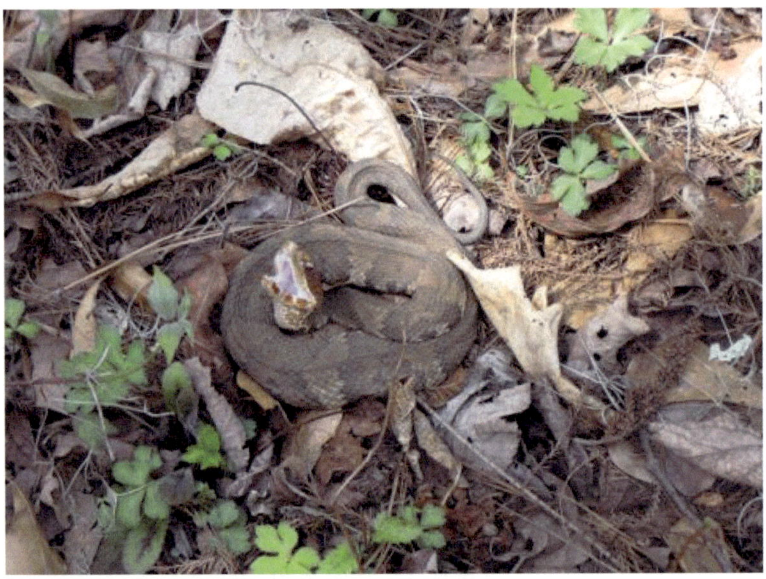

**Figure 2.**
*Adult male Eastern cottonmouth (Agkistrodon piscivorus piscivorus) from Clarendon County, South Carolina, USA. Note the gaping behavior that inspires the common name.*

as a warning to potential predators [7]. Cottonmouths occur in many of the same habitats as banded water snakes [6]. One long term mark recapture study was published by [8] for a western population of this species. Other aspects of the biology of this species have been reviewed by [6, 9].

The objective of this long-term study was to compare the ecology of syntopic populations of these semiaquatic snakes that are distantly related and from different clades [10]. *Agkistrodon piscivorus* and *Nerodia fasciata* show striking similarities and marked differences in many of their life history traits [5, 6]. Both are live bearing but differ in that *Nerodia* are income breeders with larger litters of smaller offspring whereas *Agkistrodon* are capital breeders producing small litters of larger young [11]. Female water snakes usually breed annually whereas female cottonmouths do not. Even though both species consume similar prey they employ different foraging behaviors. *Nerodia* are active foragers whereas *A. piscivorus* use sit and wait or ambush foraging [5, 12].

## 2. Methods

### 2.1 Study site

The study site was the Pee Dee Research and Education Center (PDREC), a 972 ha experimental agricultural facility owned by Clemson University, located in the upper coastal plain of Darlington County, South Carolina, USA. A series of six ponds formed by damming a creek was sampled most intensively (**Figure 3B**), a larger pond nearby was also sampled (**Figure 3A**), and Back Swamp (**Figure 3C**) an undammed creek north of the other two sites was sampled as well. All three of these wetlands flow east into Dargan's Pond which is a man-made reservoir. The ponds were surrounded by mowed grass, old field or strips of woody vegetation consisting of alder (*Alnus* sp.), willow (*Salix* sp.), loblolly pine (*Pinus taeda*), bald cypress (*Taxodium distichum*), sweet gum (*Liquidamber styraciflua*) and oaks (*Quercus* sp.). The swamp contained riparian forest which includes the above-mentioned woody plants plus red maple (*Acer rubrum*), water tupelo (*Nyssa aquatica*) and tulip poplar (*Liriodendron tulipifera*). The littoral zone of all wetlands consisted of emergent vegetation that included water lilies (*Nuphar* sp., *Nymphaea* sp.), smart weed (*Polygonum* sp.), bur-reed (*Sparganium* sp.) and patches of penny wort (*Hydrocotyle* sp.). The climate of this region consists of hot humid summers (mean June–August high temperatures during 2002–2006 were 33°C) [13]. Precipitation averaged 14.5 cm per month during June–August 2002–2006 and the region has mild winters with the mean January high temperatures of 14°C during 2002–2006.

### 2.2 Data acquisition

Snakes were sampled most frequently using double ended funnel traps although opportunistic hand captures under artificial cover objects placed along the shoreline or on or near roads were used as well. Commercially available metal minnow traps (Cuba Specialty Manufacturing Co., Filmore, NY, USA) 42 × 22 cm, plastic funnel traps (model 700; N.A.S. Incorporated, Marblehead, Ohio, USA), vinyl coated wire funnel traps (Academy Sports + Outdoors) and funnel traps made from hardware cloth that were 41 × 22 cm with 5 cm funnel openings [14] were used to sample *Nerodia fasciata* and *Agkistrodon piscivorus.* Pre-manufactured metal traps had their funnel openings enlarged to approximately 3 cm with a rake handle. Traps were placed about 3 m apart in shallow water (water depth < trap diameter) along logs, in emergent vegetation and along short aluminum drift fences. The drift

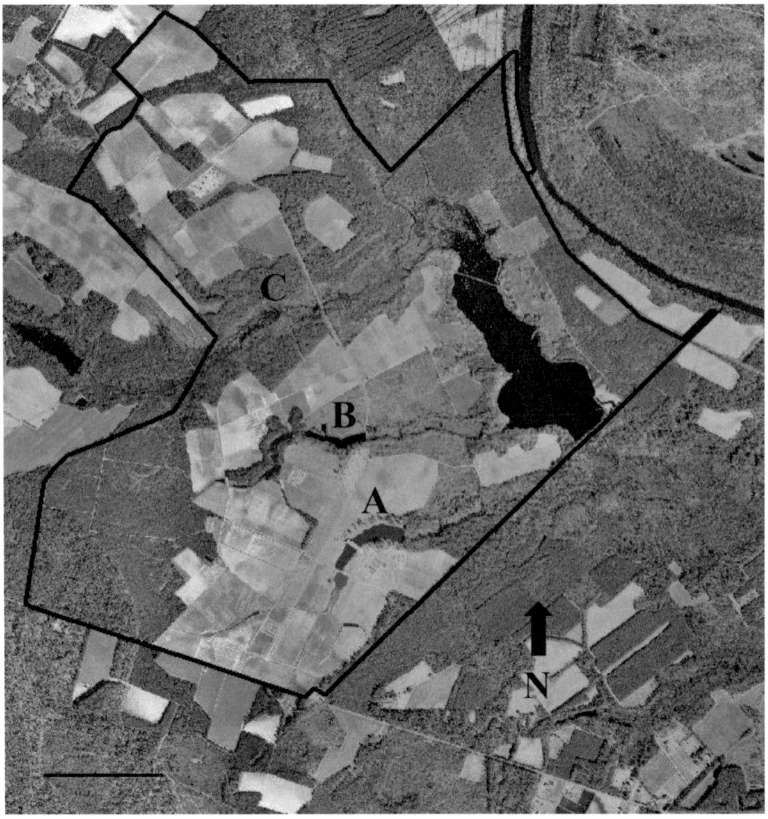


**Figure 3.**
*The Pee Dee Research and Education Center, Darlington County, South Carolina, USA. The property boundaries are outlined in black. (A) Pond near headquarters, (B) ponds where most data were collected, (C) back swamp. The Great Pee Dee River is on the upper right just outside the property boundaries. The scale bar in the lower left is 800 m.*

fences consisted of 5 m lengths of aluminum flashing oriented perpendicular to the shoreline with two traps placed at each end. Due to low capture rates, 0.007 captures/trap day (1 trap day = one trap out over 1 night, hereafter TD) in 1998 to 0.011 captures/TD in 2002, traps were checked at 48 h intervals and were either disabled or not checked on weekends when PDREC was closed. From 2010 onward traps were checked daily and closed over weekends.

Sampling took place from 1998 to 2003, 2010–2011, 2014 and 2016. Data collection from *A. piscivorus* was not started until August 1999. Sampling occurred from July–October 1998 (960 TD), May–October 1999 (4108 TD), May–July 2000 (994 TD), April–June 2001 and 2002 (810, 994 TD respectively), and May–June 2003 (757 TD) [15]. Starting in 2010 multiple shorter sampling periods per season were introduced following the robust design of [16]. Sampling occurred for 7 days in March, 11 days in April, 9 days in May–June, 9 days in August and 14 days in September during 2010. In 2011 sampling occurred for 10 days in each of May and June. During 2014 snakes were sampled for 10 days in May, 6 days in June and 5 days in September. During 2016 sampling occurred for 7 days in May and 10 days in each of June and August. The number of traps used ranged from 97 to 140. From 2010 to 2016 trapping effort ranged from 665 to 1876 TD per trapping period.

Snakes were usually processed in the field. Snout to vent length (hereafter SVL) and tail length (TL) was measured to the nearest mm with a measuring tape for *Nerodia* and a squeeze box [17] was used to measure SVL, TL, head length and head width of

*A. piscivorus*. The squeeze box was a modified plastic toolbox 66 cm × 28 cm × 28 cm. Head length and width were measured to the nearest 0.1 mm with calipers for *N. fasciata*. Mass was measured with Pesola spring scales to the nearest 1 g. Except for *Nerodia* neonates, snakes were marked with passive integrated transponder (PIT) tags [18]. Newborn *Nerodia* were marked by clipping ventral scales [19]. Sex was determined by examination of the base of the tail or by probing the tail. Data were taken from recaptures only after a minimum of 14 days had elapsed since the previous capture.

Diets were studied by examining stomach contents. Prey were palpated from the stomachs of *Nerodia* and stomach contents were recovered from cloth bags or from traps for both species. Only prey from traps with evidence of ingestion (saliva, mucous, envenomation) were included in the analyses. Prey mass was measured to the nearest 0.1 g using an electronic balance. Prey length and width were measured to the nearest 0.1 mm with calipers. Prey were identified to species when possible. Prey availability was measured by counting all prey in all traps during one day of most sampling periods. Prey counts were conducted in May and August of 2010, May of 2011, May and September of 2014 and May, June, and August of 2016 (**Table 1**). Dietary niche overlap used the formula of [20].

Females were palpated for embryos when processed. In 1999 four gravid *N. fasciata* were kept in the lab until parturition. Pregnant females were given water and food ad libitum. Food consisted of frozen/thawed fish purchased alive from a bait store. Pregnant snakes were kept on a 12:12 light: dark cycle at approximately 27°C. One died about 1 week prior to giving birth. Young were weighed and measured and marked by scale clipping. They were released at the site of maternal capture. Clutch sizes were also reported from oviductal eggs of females that died in traps. Cloacal swabs were taken from both sexes of each species from 1999 to 2001 to look for the presence of sperm. The ductus deferens of one male of each species were also examined for the presence of sperm.

Growth rates were calculated from recaptures as the difference in SVL in mm divided by the number of days between captures. The active season was considered 15 April through 15 October which is 183 days per year. Even if active the animals were considered to not be feeding and therefore not growing before 15 April or after 15 October. Negative growth values were not used in calculating growth rates and were considered the result of measurement error.

## 2.3 Statistical analyses

Tests for normality utilized the Shapiro-Wilks test and visual examination of box plots and histograms. Homoscedasticity was examined using the F-test or Bartlett's test.

| Date | Crayfish | Fishes | Amphibians | Turtles | Snakes |
|---|---|---|---|---|---|
| May 2010 | 26.6 | 53.8 | 19.4 | 0.3 | 0 |
| August 2010 | 1.9 | 88 | 9.7 | 0 | 0.4 |
| May 2011 | 20.5 | 40.5 | 38.8 | 0 | 0.2 |
| May 2014 | 24.4 | 37.2 | 38.4 | 0 | 0 |
| September 2014 | 1.6 | 72.1 | 26 | 0 | 0.3 |
| May 2016 | 22.3 | 33.7 | 43.5 | 0 | 0 |
| June 2016 | 10.8 | 28.4 | 60.6 | 0.2 | 0 |
| August 2016 | 4 | 44.2 | 48.6 | 3.1 | 0 |

**Table 1.**
*Prey availability in one pond where most snakes were sampled in this study. Numbers are percentages. See text for explanation of methods.*

Due to correlation among response variables (mass, SVL, TL, head length, head width), a multivariate analysis of variance (MANOVA) was used to test for sexual differences. The Welch t-test was used to test differences between individual variables due to unequal variances. Means are followed by ±1 standard deviation (SD) and an $\alpha \leq 0.05$ is considered significant in all statistical tests. Statistical analyses were performed in R version 4.1.1 [21]. Due to heteroscedasticity some data were natural log transformed.

## 3. Results

### 3.1 Population structure

A total of 181 *N. fasciata* and 93 *A. piscivorus* were marked in this study. Because year was used as the sampling period in the early part of this study (1998–2003) and shorter periods during the latter part of the study (2010–2016) estimates of

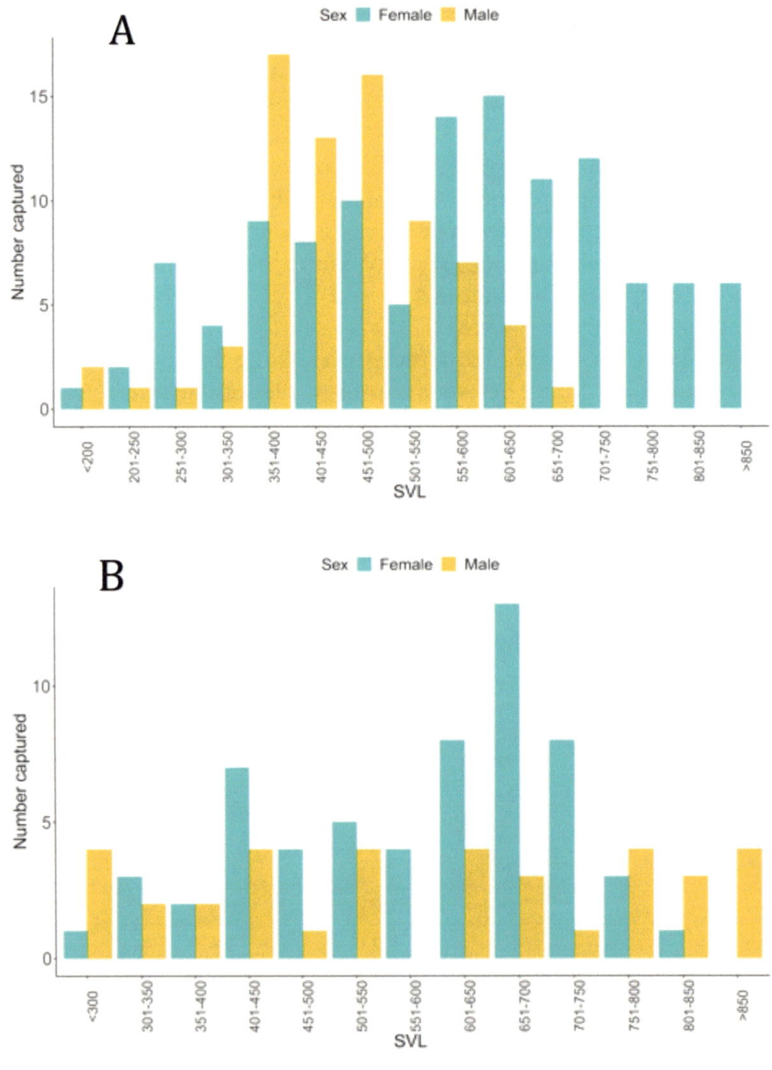


**Figure 4.**
*Size distribution of captures of each sex of (A) Nerodia fasciata; (B) Agkistrodon piscivorus at the Pee Dee Research and Education Center, Darlington County, South Carolina, USA. The ordinate is the number of captures.*

population size and survivorship could not be calculated. Recapture rates were higher for *N. fasciata* (31.5%) than for *A. piscivorus* (16%). Few neonates were captured with only 1.66% of the sample for banded water snakes and 6.45% for the cottonmouths. Subadults were defined as >1 year old but not sexually mature and made up a larger part of the sample for both species with 27% for *Nerodia* and 25.8% for *Agkistrodon*. **Figure 4A** indicates that most male *N. fasciata* were between 350 and 550 mm SVL whereas most adult females were between 550 and 750 mm SVL. There was a peak in adult female *A. piscivorus* from 600 to 750 mm SVL (**Figure 4B**). Captures of both sexes of *Nerodia* peaked in May and females showed a smaller peak in August (**Figure 5A**). Male captures gradually declined throughout the summer. Low numbers for July were due to lower trapping effort. Adult male cottonmouth captures peaked in May and declined throughout the summer (**Figure 5B**). Female captures peaked in June and showed a smaller peak in September. Sex ratios exhibited a female bias and were 1.4F:1M for each species. However, four litters of *N. fasciata* born in the lab had sex ratios that did not differ from 1:1 ($X^2$ = 4.934, df = 3, p = 0.084839).

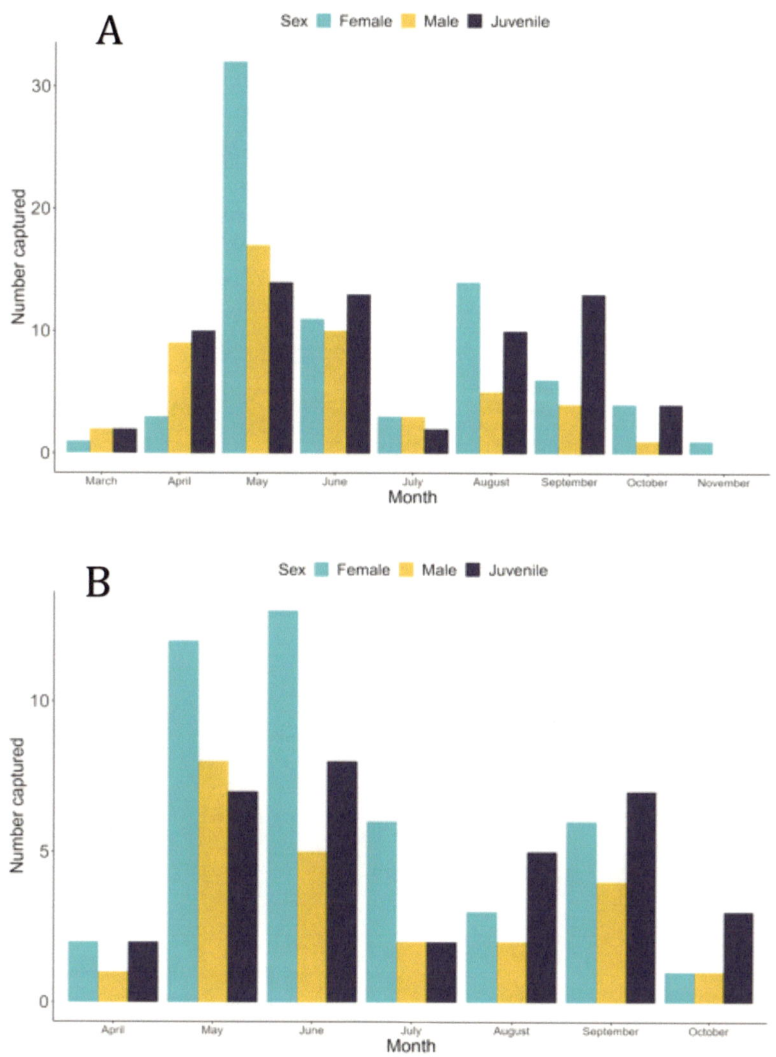


**Figure 5.**
*Seasonal distribution of captures of (A) Nerodia fasciata; (B) Agkistrodon piscivorus at the Pee Dee Research and Education Center, Darlington County, South Carolina, USA. The ordinate is the number of captures.*

Recapture latency or the time between captures in days for each species was calculated based upon an activity season from 25 March to 10 November which is 231 days per year. Mean days between captures for male *N. fasciata* were 116.5 ± 193.6 days (range 2–814 days) and for females it was 60.4 ± 58.1 days (range 4–233 days). These were not significantly different using a two-sample t-test with unequal variances ($t = -0.334$, $df = 23$, $p = 0.7415$). Mean recapture latency for both sexes combined was 80.7 ± 126.1 days (range 2–814 days). Mean recapture latency for *A. piscivorus* was 263.3 ± 575.4 days with a range of 12–2074 days. Although recapture latency was greater for *A. piscivorus* the difference was not significant ($t = -1.7025$, $df = 15.295$, $p = 0.1089$) with a two-sample t-test with unequal variances.

## 3.2 Sexual dimorphism

*Nerodia fasciata* and *Agkistrodon piscivorus* exhibit different patterns of sexual size dimorphism. Females are larger in *N. fasciata* whereas males are larger in *A. piscivorus* (**Table 2**). A multivariate analysis of variance (MANOVA) showed significant differences between the sexes for *N. fasciata* (Pillais' trace = 0.340, $F(1, 140) = 14.002$, $p < 0.001$) for the morphological variables in **Table 2** but not for *A. piscivorus* (Pillais' trace = 0.117, $F(1, 86) = 2.17$, $p = 0.065$). Female *N. fasciata* were significantly greater in mass ($t = 3.5508$, $p = 0.0005$), SVL ($t = 3.983$, $p = 0.0001$), head length ($t = 5.025$, $p < 0.001$) and head width ($t = 5.218$, $p < 0.001$). However, tail length was not significantly different ($t = 1.6743$, $p = 0.0963$) between males and females. Relative tail length (tail length/total length; hereafter RTL) was greater for males of both species. For *N. fasciata* mean male RTL = 0.262 ± 0.016 (0.197–0.286, N = 55) whereas females averaged 0.241 ± 0.014 (0.197–0.269, N = 87). Values

| | *Nerodia fasciata* | | *Agkistrodon piscivorus* | |
|---|---|---|---|---|
| | **Males** | **Females** | **Males** | **Females** |
| Mass (g) | 129.3 ± 58.2 | 340.8 ± 165.7 | 518 ± 305 | 412.9 ± 147.3 |
| Range | 54–307 | 131–730 | 165–1316 | 125–814 |
| N | 42 | 55 | 22 | 36 |
| Snout vent length (mm) | 504.5 ± 73.9 | 670.1 ± 98 | 731.3 ± 139.6 | 650.5 ± 85.2 |
| Range | 397–655 | 505–915 | 500–980 | 490–848 |
| N | 42 | 57 | 22 | 36 |
| Tail length (mm) | 178.1 ± 25.4 | 210.4 ± 28.4 | 130.5 ± 26.9 | 116.6 ± 15.4 |
| Range | 143–230 | 163–266 | 96–175 | 80–151 |
| N | 31 | 36 | 20 | 35 |
| Head length (mm) | 28 ± 4.3 | 37.4 ± 5.5 | 43.9 ± 5.8 | 41.8 ± 4.9 |
| Range | 18.5–37.3 | 24.2–51.3 | 34–51.5 | 32–48 |
| N | 42 | 57 | 22 | 36 |
| Head width (mm) | 15.8 ± 3.4 | 22.7 ± 3.8 | 37 ± 5.9 | 37.3 ± 4.2 |
| Range | 10.8–29.5 | 15.7–31.5 | 25.1–48.5 | 27.9–44 |
| N | 42 | 57 | 22 | 36 |

**Table 2.**
*Sexual dimorphism in body and head size of adult Nerodia fasciata and Agkistrodon piscivorus from South Carolina, USA. Numbers are means ±1 standard deviation.*

for male *A. piscivorus* were 0.159 ± 0.019 (0.111–0.229, N = 33) and for females 0.153 ± 0.016 (0.110–0.197, N = 56). The sexual dichromatism with males retaining a bolder banding pattern was also observed in this population of *A. piscivorus* [22].

### 3.3 Growth rates

Growth rate estimates were available for 28 *N. fasciata* and 6 *A. piscivorus*. Growth rates (mean ± 1 SD) were 0.726 ± 0.626 mm/day (0–2.3 mm/day) for *N. fasciata* and 0.783 ± 1.26 mm/day (0.029–3.31 mm/day) for *A. piscivorus*. Mean female *N. fasciata* growth rates were almost twice that of males (female 0.824 ± 0.672 mm/day, 0–2.3 mm/day, N = 21; male 0.432 ± 0.353, 1–1.029 mm/day, N = 7). Small sample size precluded statistical analysis. One female *A. piscivorus* that was originally marked on 3 May 2001 was recaptured on 28 April 2010 and had grown only 52 mm in almost 9 years and had a growth rate of 0.0322 mm/day.

### 3.4 Food habits

Both species fed frequently upon fishes whereas banded water snakes ate amphibians frequently but not reptiles and cottonmouths consumed reptiles but few amphibians (**Table 3**). The number of prey per stomach ranged from 1 to 8 for *N. fasciata* and 1–5 for *A. piscivorus*. Multiple prey were found in 10 of 24 (41.7%) banded water snakes and 3 of 5 (60%) cottonmouths. One 715 mm SVL female *A. piscivorus* contained 1 catfish, 1 sunfish (*Lepomis* sp.), 1 pickerel (*Esox* sp.), 1 frog (*Lithobates* sp.) and one Eastern musk turtle (*Sternotherus odoratus*). All but the turtle was swallowed headfirst. Mass ratios (prey mass/snake mass) given as mean ± 1 standard deviation followed by the range was greater for *A. piscivorus* (0.159 ± 0.208, 0.186–0.526) than for *N. fasciata* (0.109 ± 0.083, 0.0096–0.3889). Banded water snake stomach contents were 44% fishes and 56% amphibians whereas cottonmouth stomach contents were 46% fishes, 50% reptiles and 4% amphibians. Only one *N. fasciata,* a female 380 mm SVL, had eaten one Eastern mosquito fish (*Gambusia holbrooki*). Larval anurans made up the largest proportion of amphibians, with metamorphosed anurans contributing 18.7% and salamanders only 1.7% of the total. The dietary niche overlap [20] was low between these two species (O = 0.01024). Only *A. piscivorus* more than 550 mm SVL included reptiles in their diets and *N. fasciata* over 750 mm SVL dropped amphibians from their diets. Banded water snakes did not swallow prey headfirst more frequently than tail first ($X^2$ = 0.34, df = 1, $p > 0.05$) however, fishes were swallowed headfirst significantly more often, and amphibians tail first (2 × 2 contingency table, $X^2$ = 17.049, df = 1, $p < 0.05$). Small sample sizes precluded statistical analysis of *A. piscivorus* stomach contents.

Prey availability was assessed by counting all potential prey in the traps during one day per sampling period. There were eight prey censuses during this study (**Table 1**). Crayfish decreased in abundance during the season. Fishes and amphibians varied between sampling dates but did not show any discernible trends. *Gambusia holbrooki* made up a mean of 11.13 ± 7.73% (1.6–23.7%) of the samples.

### 3.5 Reproduction

The smallest male *N. fasciata* with sperm in the cloaca was 397 mm SVL and was sampled on 24 September 1999. Because a specimen 395 mm SVL sampled on 28 June 1999 lacked cloacal sperm, 400 mm SVL was designated as adult size for male *N. fasciata*. Eight males contained sperm (397–600 mm SVL) and 8 others (320–655 mm SVL) did not. Two males with sperm were from May, 4 from June

| Prey category | *Nerodia fasciata* | *Agkistrodon piscivorus* |
|---|---|---|
| | N (%) | N (%) |
| Cyprinidae | 1 (1.7) | 1 (4.3) |
| *Cyprinella* sp. | | 1 (4.3) |
| Ictaluridae | 1 (1.7) | 1 (4.3) |
| *Noturus* sp. | 1 (1.7) | |
| Esocidae | | |
| *Esox americanus* | 2 (3.4) | |
| *Esox niger* | | 1 (4.3) |
| *Esox* sp. | 3 (5.1) | 3 (13) |
| Poeciliidae | | |
| *Gambusia holbrooki* | 1 (1.7) | |
| Centrarchidae | 1 (1.7) | |
| *Enneacanthus* sp. | 1 (1.7) | |
| *Lepomis punctatus* | 1 (1.7) | |
| *Lepomis* sp. | 7 (11.9) | 2 (8.7) |
| *Micropterus salmoides* | 1 (1.7) | |
| Unidentifiable fish | 7 (11.9) | 1 (4.3) |
| Sirenidae | | |
| *Siren intermedia* | 1 (1.7) | |
| Hylidae | | |
| *Hyla cinerea* | 1 (1.7) | |
| Ranidae | | |
| *Lithobates catesbeianus* | 5 (8.5) | |
| *Lithobates sphenocephalus* | 1 (1.7) | |
| *Lithobates* sp. | 4 (6.8) | 1 (4.3) |
| *Lithobates* larvae | 20 (33.9) | |
| Kinosternidae | | |
| *Sternotherus odoratus* | | 1 (4.3) |
| Colubridae | | |
| *Nerodia fasciata* | | 11 (47.8) |
| Total prey | 59 | 23 |

**Table 3.**
*Frequency of occurrence of prey found in 25 Nerodia fasciata and 14 Agkistrodon piscivorus from the Pee Dee Research and Education Center, Darlington County, South Carolina, USA. N is the number of prey items in the sample.*

and 2 from September. The males lacking sperm included 4 from May, 1 from June, 2 from July and 1 from August. The smallest male *A. piscivorus* that had sperm in the ductus deferens was 500 mm SVL and was caught on 26 May 2000. Another male (863 mm SVL) had cloacal sperm on 23 May. Three males lacking sperm were 768–961 mm SVL and were sampled in May (2) and July.

The smallest gravid female *N. fasciata* was 575 mm SVL however 500 mm SVL was used as the size for sexual maturity in analyses [23]. In 2000 92% of females were gravid and 91% in 2006 indicating that most females probably reproduce annually in this population. Only 58% of female *A. piscivorus* were gravid in 2000 indicating a likely biennial reproduction in females of this species. The smallest gravid female *A. piscivorus* was 660 mm SVL and 500 mm SVL was used as minimum adult size for females of this species as well [24]. During 1999 four gravid *N. fasciata* were brought into the lab until parturition. One specimen died on 13 August with embryos in developmental stage 36 [25]. Clutch sizes ranged from 12 to 28 (mean ± 1 SD) was 18.45 ± 5.24 (N = 11). There was a significant positive correlation between maternal SVL and clutch size (r = 0.723, p = 0.018, N = 10). Dates of parturition for females that gave birth in the lab were 5 and 23 August and 3 September. The earliest in the season that females were found to be pregnant was 17 May for *N. fasciata* and 18 May for *A. piscivorus*. Relative clutch mass (RCM) ranged from 0.19–0.478 (mean ± 1 SD) was 0.335 ± 0.119 (N = 4). Mean neonate mass from three litters born in the lab was 3.89 ± 0.51 g (3–5 g, N = 66) and the mean SVL for these same snakes was 153.72 ± 5.77 mm (133–166, N = 66). Data on size of oviductal eggs came from four females collected in late May and early June which were at a similar enough developmental stage to be lumped into a single data set. Mean oviductal egg length was 21.30 ± 5.01 mm (13.2–32.7 mm, N = 66 ova) and mean oviductal egg width for the same ova was 13.82 ± 3.99 mm (7.7–19.9 mm, N = 66). One 715 mm SVL *A. piscivorus* collected on 26 May 2000 contained five oviductal eggs with a mean length of 35.68 ± 1.63 mm (33.9–37.5 mm) and a mean width of 21.94 ± 0.82 mm (21.0–22.9 mm). Three *N. fasciata* with oviductal eggs had more in the right oviduct than in the left. Mean (± 1SD) for the right oviduct was 10.33 ± 1.15 (9–11) and for the left 7 ± 1 (6–8) but not significantly more ($X^2$ = 1.924, df 1, p > 0.05). No banded water snakes had more in the left oviduct and the one *A. piscivorus* had two in the right oviduct and three in the left.

Stub tails and body scars can give information on potential predation pressure on snakes [26]. Nineteen male *N. fasciata* exhibited stub tails (15) or body scarring (4) which was 35% of the sample. Female *N. fasciata* showed 37.6% injured snakes with 26 of 32 with stub tails and 6 with body scarring. Cottonmouths showed a much lower frequency of injuries with only 4 of 32 males (12.5%) showing injuries and only one with body scarring. Females had the same numbers of injuries which showed an 8.3% injury rate.

## 4. Discussion

### 4.1 Population structure

Because population sizes and survival rates could not be estimated the discussion of population structure will focus on age structure and sex ratios. Only 3 neonate *N. fasciata* and 6 neonate *A. piscivorus* were caught in this study. Under sampling of juvenile snakes is usually attributed to low survival rates [27] however it may also be from trapping bias as neonatal snakes can escape through the mesh of traps [28] which I think may have occurred in this study for *N. fasciata*. Neonatal *A. piscivorus* are too large to escape through the trap mesh. Captures of subadult snakes, defined as >1 year old but not sexually mature, were frequent for both species (**Figure 4**). This finding may indicate these populations have a relatively young age structure and therefor may be undergoing population growth [29].

Sex ratios for both species were skewed in favor of females which I think may be due to sampling bias. Primary sex ratios were not different from unity for *N. fasciata*. There was a secondary peak of captures of postparturent females in August (**Figure 4**). Sometimes the same females were caught in the same traps on consecutive days (J. Camper, unpublished observation) as found by [30] in another South

Carolina population. Female capture bias was shown by [31] for both focal species in Texas. In another study in Texas, using a different sampling method, [8] found a sex ratio not significantly different from one for *A. piscivorus*. Three other populations of this species were found to have slight male bias [22, 32, 33] as did one study of *N. fasciata* in another region of South Carolina [32].

### 4.2 Sexual dimorphism

I found that female *N. fasciata* were significantly greater in mass, SVL and head size than males whereas tail length was not significantly different. Similar results were found in another South Carolina *N. fasciata* population located about 180 km southwest of my study site [32]. The latter study did not examine head size, however. Patterns of sexual dimorphism in *A. piscivorus* contrasted with *N. fasciata* but were not statistically significant and in agreement with [22, 34]. Although head size was not significantly different between the sexes of cottonmouths [33] found that males had longer quadrate bones than females. The males in this population retain a bold banding pattern similar to juveniles that was first documented by [22]. Relative tail length averaged about 2% longer in males of *N. fasciata* but less than 1% longer in *A. piscivorus.* Similar findings for both species were published by [35] for specimens collected from throughout North Carolina. The values reported here were higher for *Nerodia* but close to those of *Agkistrodon* calculated by [34].

### 4.3 Growth rates

Growth rates have not been reported for *N. fasciata* so they will be compared to the closely related *Nerodia sipedon* [10]. Growth rates from this population were higher than the 0.12 mm/day mean for male and the 0.14 mm/day mean for female *N. sipedon* in Lake Erie [26]. The *N. sipedon* study was from a northern population with a much shorter growing season which could affect growth rates. Three neonate *N. fasciata* caught in August (1 snake) and September (2) averaged 173.67 ± 16.29 mm SVL. This was 20 mm longer than the mean for lab born snakes suggesting that growth may occur before their first winter. Cottonmouth growth rates reported here were also higher than reported for western populations of 0.210–0.280 mm/day [24] and 0.170–0.434 mm/day [8]. Because male *N. fasciata* mature at about 400 mm SVL (see below) they may reach sexual maturity by the end of their second year and mate the following spring. Females probably mature 1 year later when they surpass 500 mm SVL. Based upon these growth rates, male *A. piscivorus* may reach sexual maturity in about 2.5 years and females in about 4 years.

### 4.4 Food habits

These two species exhibited little dietary niche overlap which was probably due to *A. piscivorus* having few amphibians and many reptiles in its diet. The banded water snake diet documented in this population is similar to that found in other populations [5, 36] except that *G. holbrooki* was consumed only once by one juvenile banded water snake. In a study in Louisiana *N. fasciata* consumed 30.6% *G. holbrooki* and 11.2% amphibians [37]. *Nerodia fasciata* may be avoiding *G. holbrooki* at this study site because it appears to be an abundant species at this locality and only one specimen was found in the stomach contents. Banded water snakes ingested significantly more fish headfirst. This could be due to scales covering the fish. Snakes feeding on reptiles usually swallow prey headfirst and scales are used in prey orientation [38, 39]. *Agkistrodon piscivorus* is known for its broad diet that includes mammals, birds and their eggs, alligators and pit vipers in addition to what was found in this study [6, 40]. Five different species of amphibians were found in North Carolina specimens [35]. There is geographic variation in the diet of this species also, as evidenced by [41] finding no amphibians in the diet to amphibians making a large proportion of the diet in other populations [24, 33]. No novel prey were found in the diet of *A. piscivorus* in this study but the lesser siren (*Siren intermedia*) is a newly documented prey species for *N. fasciata.* Larger mass ratios for *A. piscivorus* as compared to *N. fasciata* was not surprising given that the former have relatively larger heads and a greater gape [33].

Frequencies of stub tails and body scarring were more than 20% higher in *N. fasciata* than in *A. piscivorus* at my study site. Injury frequency may reflect predation intensity or predator efficiency [26]. I believe the former to be true in this study because of the relatively high frequency in *N. fasciata* and the lower frequency in *A. piscivorus*. Because the latter is a large pit viper with potent venom it probably experiences less predation pressure than *N. fasciata*. Injury frequency was about 15% higher for *N. fasciata* in this study when compared to another population about 180 km to the southwest [34].

### 4.5 Reproduction

Litter sizes documented here agree with what has been found in other populations of both species [24, 32, 35, 41–46]. The correlation of maternal SVL and litter size is well documented in snakes [47] and was found for another South Carolina population of *N. fasciata* [32]. The RCM found in this study is larger than the 0.201 reported for one specimen of *N. fasciata* [48]. Parturition dates for *N. fasciata* were like those in other populations [43, 45]. Neonate sizes reported here averaged 4 mm SVL longer than reported by [28] for another South Carolina population. Three neonates trapped in August and September were small enough to escape through the trap mesh [28]. The mean SVL for 6 neonate *A. piscivorus* trapped in this study was 277.67 ± 56.46 (215–344) which is larger than reported for other populations [8, 24, 42] but smaller than neonates from Florida [49]. The low proportion of pregnant female *A. piscivorus* found here suggests that females give birth biennially in this population. Most populations of cottonmouths reproduce biennially [8, 24, 49, 50]. However, some populations may have annual reproduction [23, 42]. All three gravid female banded water snakes had more ova in the right oviduct which was also reported by [51] for one Texas specimen. More embryos in the right oviduct of *A. piscivorus* were also reported by [44, 46] unlike what was found here.

## 5. Conclusions

Two common snake species, the banded water snake (*Nerodia fasciata*) and the Eastern cottonmouth (*Agkistrodon piscivorus*) were studied on the coastal plain of southeastern North America. This long-term mark-recapture study used funnel traps to sample the snakes. Approximately 180 *N. fasciata* and 93 *A. piscivorus* were marked in this study. Recapture frequencies were low and population size estimates and survival rates could not be calculated.

Sexual size dimorphism favors females in *N. fasciata* which were significantly larger in mass, SVL and head size than males. Males were the larger sex for *A. piscivorus* but this was not significant. Growth rates were 0.726 ± 0.626 mm/day (0–2.3 mm/day) for *N. fasciata* and 0.783 ± 1.26 mm/day (0.029–3.31 mm/day) for *A. piscivorus*. Both species exhibited female biased secondary sex ratios which may be due to sampling bias. Primary sex ratios of four litters of *N. fasciata* were not significantly different from one.

Male *N. fasciata* reach sexual maturity at about 400 mm SVL and females at about 500 mm SVL. Males may be able to reach this length in about 2 years and females in 3 years. Male *A. piscivorus* reach maturity at 450 to 500 mm SVL which takes about 3 years. Female *A. piscivorus* mature at about 500 to 550 mm SVL which probably takes 3–4 years.

Both species fed upon fish and *N. fasciata* included many amphibians in its diet whereas *A. piscivorus* ate reptiles but few amphibians. Fish prey were swallowed headfirst and amphibian prey usually tail first. Female banded water snakes appear to breed annually whereas female cottonmouths probably breed every other year. Clutch sizes ranged from 12 to 28 with a mean of 18.45 ± 5.24 (N = 11) for *N. fasciata*. There was a significant positive correlation between maternal SVL and clutch size. One female *A. piscivorus* contained 5 oviductal eggs. Clearly more work is needed on these populations to determine population size estimates, survivorship and to elucidate the reproductive biology of *A. piscivorus.*

## Acknowledgements

Funding was provided by Francis Marion University (FMU) and the South Carolina Governor's School of Science and Mathematics (GSSM). The administration of the Pee Dee Research and Education Center graciously provided access to the property. The South Carolina Department of Natural Resources provided scientific collecting permits. Jason Doll helped with statistical analysis. Numerous FMU students helped with field work including J.R. Burger, L.D. Chick, A. Crawford, M.P. Grooms, R. Hanson, T. Hardymon, M. Jaco, T. Jensen, A. MacNeil, B. Reid, H. Sellers, and T. Tedder. GSSM students M. Blew, M. Chandler and M. Patel also aided in field work. Ben Camper helped in the field as well. This research benefitted greatly by discussions with J.D. Willson.

## Author details

Jeffrey D. Camper
Department of Biology, Francis Marion University, Florence, South Carolina, USA

*Address all correspondence to: jcamper@fmarion.edu

## References

[1] Herron J, Freeman S. Evolutionary Analysis. 5th ed. New York, New York, USA: Pearson; 2014. p. 850

[2] Seigel R. Summary: Future research on snakes, or how to combat lizard envy. In: Seigel R, Collins T, editors. Snakes—Ecology and Behavior. New York, New York, USA: McGraw-Hill; 1993. pp. 395-402

[3] Reinert H. Habitat selection in snakes. In: Seigel R, Collins T, editors. Snakes—Ecology and Behavior. McGraw-Hill; 1993. pp. 201-240

[4] Peterson C, Gibson A, Dorcas M. Snake thermal ecology: The causes and consequences of body-temperature variation. In: Seigel R, Collins T, editors. Snakes—Ecology and Behavior. McGraw-Hill; 1993. pp. 241-314

[5] Gibbons J, Dorcas M. North American Watersnakes: A Natural History. Norman, Oklahoma, USA: University of Oklahoma; 2004. p. 438

[6] Ernst C, Ernst M. Snakes of the United States and Canada. Washington, DC, USA: Smithsonian; 2003. p. 668

[7] Camper J. The Reptiles of South Carolina. University of South Carolina; 2019. p. 273

[8] Ford N. Ecology of the western cottonmouth (*Agkistrodon piscivorus leucostoma*) in northeastern Texas. In: Schuett G, Höggren M, Douglas M, Greene H, editors. Biology of the Vipers. Eagle Mountain, Utah, USA: Eagle Mountain Publishing; 2002. pp. 167-177

[9] Gloyd H. In: Conant R, editor. Snakes of the *Agkistrodon* Complex. A Monographic Review. Oxford, Ohio, USA: Thomas Shore; 1990. p. 614

[10] Pyron R, Burbrink F, Wiens J. A phylogeny and revised classification of Squamata, including 4161 species of lizards and snakes. BMC Evolutionary Biology. 2013;**13**:93. DOI: 10.1186/1471-2148-13-93

[11] Bonnet X, Bradshaw D, Shine R. Capital versus income breeding: An ectothermic perspective. Oikos. 1998;**83**:333-342

[12] Eskew E, Willson J, Winne C. Ambush site selection and ontogenetic shifts in foraging strategy in a semi-aquatic pit viper, the Eastern cottonmouth. Journal of Zoology. 2009;**277**:179-186. DOI: 10.1111/j.1469-7998.2009.00527.x

[13] Camper J, Chick D. Seasonal variation in the spatial ecology of the banded watersnake (*Nerodia fasciata fasciata*). Herpetologica. 2010;**66**: 464-475

[14] Fitch H. Collecting and life history techniques. In: Seigel R, Collins T, Novak S, editors. Snakes: Ecology and Evolutionary Biology. New York, New York, USA: MacMillan; 1987. pp. 143-164

[15] Camper J. Observations on problems with using funnel traps to sample aquatic snakes. Herpetological Review. 2005;**36**:288-290

[16] Pollock K. A capture-recapture design robust to unequal probability of capture. Journal of Wildlife Management. 1982; **46**:752-757

[17] Bertram N, Larsen K. Putting the squeeze on venomous snakes: Accuracy and precision of length measurements take with the "squeeze box". Herpetological Review. 2004;**35**:235-238

[18] Camper J, Dixon J. Evaluation of a Microchip Marking System for Amphibians and Reptiles. Vol. 7100-159. Austin, Texas, USA: Texas Parks and

Wildlife Department: Research Publication; 1988. pp. 1-22

[19] Brown W, Parker W. A ventral scale clipping system for permanently marking snakes (Reptilia, Serpentes). Journal of Herpetology. 1976;**10**:247-249

[20] Pianka E. The structure of lizard communities. Annual Review of Ecology and Systematics. 1973;**4**:53-74

[21] R Core Team. R: A language and environment for statistical computing. Vienna Austria: R Foundation for Statistical Computing; 2021. Available from: http://www.R-project.org

[22] Zaidan F III. Western cottonmouth (*Agkistrodon piscivorus leucostoma*) sexual dimorphism and dichromatism in northwestern Arkansas. Herpetological Natural History. 2001;**8**:79-82

[23] Kofron C. Reproduction of aquatic snakes in south-central Louisiana. Herpetologica. 1979;**35**:44-50

[24] Burkett R. Natural History of Cottonmouth Moccasin, *Agkistrodon piscivorus* (Reptilia). Vol. 17. University of Kansas Museum of Natural History; 1966. pp. 435-491

[25] Zehr D. Stages in the normal development of the common garter snake, *Thamnophis sirtalis sirtalis*. Copeia. 1962:322-329

[26] King R. Populational ecology of the Lake Erie water snake, *Nerodia sipedon insularum*. Copeia. 1986:757-772

[27] Parker W, Plummer M. Population ecology. In: Seigel R, Collins T, Novak S, editors. Snakes: Ecology and Evolutionary Biology. MacMillan; 1987. pp. 253-301

[28] Willson J, Winne C, Keck M. Empirical tests of biased body size distributions in aquatic snake captures. Copeia. 2008:401-408. DOI: 10.1643/CH-07-035

[29] Pianka E. Evolutionary Ecology. 5th ed. New York, New York, USA: Harper Collins; 1994. p. 486

[30] Willson J, Winne C, Todd B. Ecological and methodological factors affecting detectability and population estimation in elusive species. Journal of Wildlife Management. 2011;**75**:36-45

[31] Keck M. A new technique for sampling semi-aquatic snake populations. Herpetological Natural History. 1994;**2**:101-103

[32] Semlitsch R, Gibbons J. Body size dimorphism and sexual selection in two species of water snakes. Copeia. 1982:974-976

[33] Vincent S, Herrel A, Irschick D. Sexual dimorphism in head shape and diet in the cottonmouth snake (*Agkistrodon piscivorus*). Journal of Zoology London. 2004;**264**:53-59. DOI: 10.1017/S0952836904005503

[34] Kaufman G, Gibbons J. Weight-length relationships in thirteen species of snakes in the southeastern United States. Herpetologica. 1975;**31**:31-37

[35] Palmer W, Braswell A. Reptiles of North Carolina. Univ North Carolina Press; 1995. p. 412

[36] Durso A, Willson J, Winne C. Habitat influences diet overlap in aquatic snake assemblages. Journal of Zoology. 2013;**291**:185-193. DOI: 10.1111/jzo.12061

[37] Mushinsky H, Hebrard J. Food partitioning by five species of water snakes in Louisiana. Herpetologica. 1977;**33**:162-166

[38] Camper J, Dixon J. Food habits of three species of striped whipsnakes, *Masticophis* (Serpentes: Colubridae). Texas Journal of Science. 2000;**52**: 83-92

[39] Greene H. Feeding behavior and diet of the Eastern coral snake, *Micrurus fulvius*. In: Seigel R, Hunt L, Knight J, Malaret L, Zuschlag N, editors. Vertebrate Ecology and Systematics: A Tribute to Henry S. Fitch. Lawrence, Kansas, USA: University of Kansas; 1984. pp. 147-162

[40] Kofron C. Foods and habitats of aquatic snakes (Reptilia, Serpentes) in a Louisiana swamp. Journal of Herpetology. 1978;**12**:543-554

[41] Wharton C. The cottonmouth moccasin on Sea Horse Key, Florida. Bulletin of the Florida State Museum. 1969;**14**:227-272

[42] Blem C. Reproduction of the Eastern cottonmouth *Agkistrodon piscivorus piscivorus* (Serpentes: Viperidae) at the Northern edge of its range. Brimleyana. 1981;**5**:117-128

[43] Ford N, Cobb V, Lamar W. Reproductive data on snakes from northeastern Texas. Texas Journal of Science. 1990;**42**:355-368

[44] Tinkle D. Observation of reptiles and amphibians in a Louisiana swamp. American Midland Naturalist. 1959;**62**:189-205

[45] Clark R. Snakes of the hill parishes of Louisiana. Journal of the Tennessee Academy of Science. 1949;**24**:244-261

[46] Allen E, Swindell D. Cottonmouth moccasin of Florida. Herpetologica. 1948;**4**:1-16

[47] Seigel R, Ford N. Reproductive ecology. In: Seigel R, Collins T, Novak S, editors. Snakes: Ecology and Evolutionary Biology. New York, New York, USA: MacMillan; 1987. pp. 210-252

[48] Seigel R, Fitch H. Ecological patterns of relative clutch mass in snakes. Oecologia. 1984;**61**:293-301

[49] Wharton C. Reproduction and growth in the cottonmouths, *Agkistrodon piscivorus* Lacépède, of Cedar Keys, Florida. Copeia. 1966:149-161

[50] Scott D, Fischer R, Congdon J, Busa S. Whole body lipid dynamics and reproduction in the Eastern Cottonmouth, *Agkistrodon piscivorus*. Herpetologica. 1995;**51**:472-487

[51] Kennedy J. Natural history notes on some snakes of Eastern Texas. Texas Journal of Science. 1964;**16**:210-215